life in flow

Inspiration, sequences
and poses to bring yoga
into your everyday life

KATE KENDALL

MURDOCH BOOKS

SYDNEY · LONDON

Contents

Introduction

Written with a whole heart, *Life in Flow* is intended to be a useful, sincere and contemporary guide to living your yoga on and off the mat: to embracing joy, creating more meaningful relationships and discovering your true life's calling.

This book is for the yoga and mindfulness curious as well as for those who have already begun their spiritual journey and are craving real-world tools and everyday rituals for living in an aligned way off the mat.

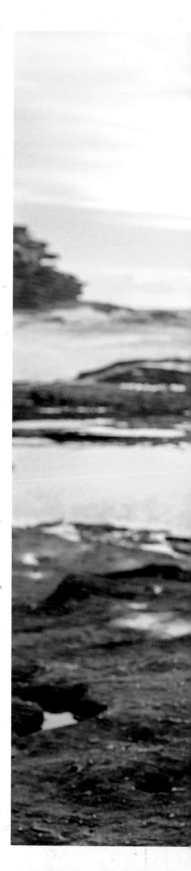

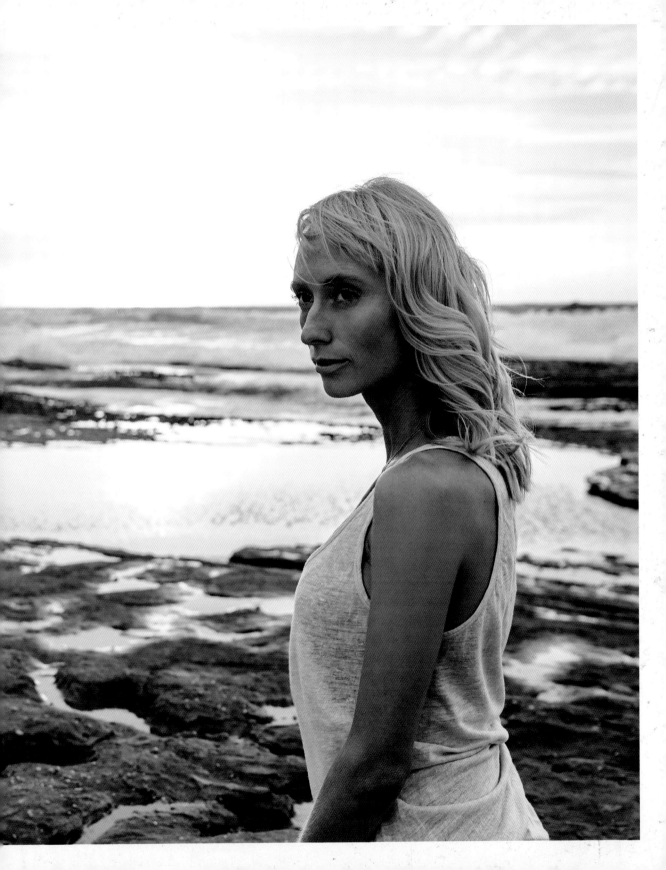

The four sections of the book provide guidance and tips for slowing down, embracing joy, creating more conscious connections and remembering that when we are in service to others, life feels not only more rewarding, but fulfilling and whole.

The book also brings ancient yogic philosophies into a modern-day light, borrowing inspiration from Buddhist and Hindu traditions. I am passionate about learning and putting into practice both traditions. Many aspects have useful applications for today's world. We can lean into the symbolism behind the deities as well as the gentle suggestions for living discovered in the eight limbs of yoga, which are all steeped in the Hindu tradition. And we can practise 'being' the compassion and change we wish to see in the world, as embodied in the Buddhist tradition.

The illustrated Moving Meditations you will see in the book are flavoured with the theme of each section and are intended to make you feel good as well as help you experience meditation through movement.

By bringing my own experiences into this book, and highlighting friends who

I consider to be 'in flow', I intend to give you useful tips and tools for greeting stress and anxiety, as well as real-life examples of how, when you learn to slow down, reprioritise, follow your heart and be in service to others, remarkable things come your way. There is no exception to this. It's a universal truth – as I like to say, these things will come your way 'only always'.

You see, as far as the yogi is concerned, life's about finding a balance between hustle and heart: cultivating joy while also making space for grief and sadness; connecting with others while connecting to self; and giving to others just as you give to yourself. This is what we call wholehearted living – being open to the whole range of human emotions and experiences.

And when we can find that sweet spot that sits between the ends and be open to the experiences that are in front of us in any one moment, life gets sweeter.

To live your yoga, or 'own your flow', is to be 'all in' and totally up for this ride we call life, skimming over nothing and feeling everything; to greet the world around us with an open, playful and curious heart.

Life's about finding an even flow – not holding onto anything too rigidly and being willing to let go when something has run its course. Impermanence is one of our greatest life lessons and when we can strike a balance between holding on and letting go, we allow ourselves to step back into the flow of life, which is always changing. It might seem scary at first but if we start to 'ride' the flow, it takes us on epic journeys that would have been unknown to us had we held rigidly to what felt comfortable. This flow of life 'only always' knows which way to go. You don't have to know. It's called trust.

But how can we be in flow and fully trust if we're running at a frantic pace, always striving to get ahead?

If we really want to live life fully and wholeheartedly, we must first learn to slow down, savour our moments and make choices that are aligned to our greatest good. I know that when I'm at my busiest, I tend to forget what's really important to me. But if I can slow down for long enough to remember, I reprioritise and reset. I'm back. It doesn't mean we have to run at a slow pace forever; laziness is not what this is about (there are definitely times to hustle). It's just a prompt to remember what's important and move forward from there.

In a fast-paced, busy world, the centuries-old philosophies and traditions of yoga are applicable now more than ever and so here they are, delivered in a friendly, light-hearted and easy-to-digest way.

This book is an ode to the true meaning of yoga – coming from the Sanskrit root *yuj* or *yug*, which essentially means 'yoke' – which is to unite or connect. It's a book less about 'self-help' and more about 'helping others' and strengthening relationships and community.

I hope you find this book both practical and inspiring and that it fills you with faith to follow the charm and do what lights you up. Because yoga is all about listening; listening to your body's natural rhythms, listening to the gradual pull of the universe and listening (caringly) to each other.

How we do one thing is how we do all.

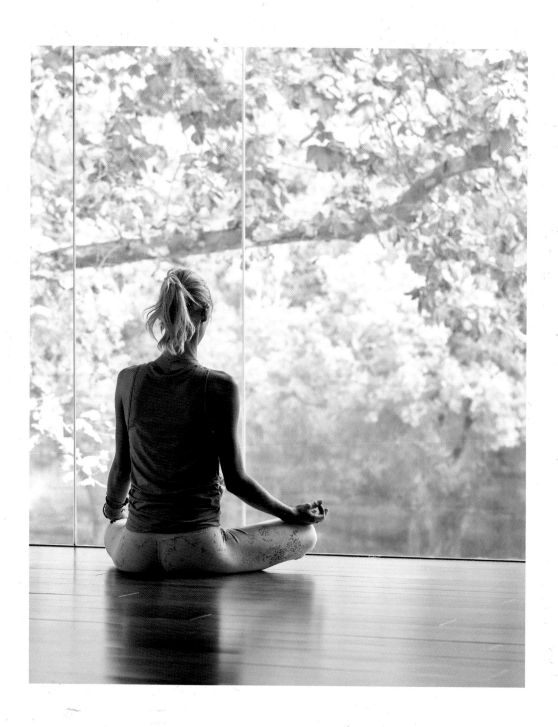

What is 'living in flow'?

And how it took a big mess for me to find it.

I guess you could say the message in this book comes from a messy time of my life when I was completely burnt out; a time when I played the victim for way too long and blamed everyone and everything but myself for having no control over my energy levels, let alone my life or direction.

Let me take you back to sunny Bondi, where my yogic journey began. I'd just come back from a year-long stint in the UK where I'd done nothing but drink, party and play. Sounds fun, and it was, but in hindsight it didn't do me any good. I wasn't in the right headspace. You see, I'd been on anti-depressants for some time and all that overindulgence was messing with me.

My experience of depression was like this: I'd walk around in a fog, skimming over experiences and not feeling much. And feeling is the whole point.

It's what makes us insanely, beautifully and imperfectly, perfectly human.

I felt a constant state of dullness. It was as if I was walking around with my head in fog, not knowing why I felt the urge to cry or what was wrong with me. And when I was put on anti-depressants during my university days, I just figured that this was how I would cope for the rest of my life. It didn't occur to me that I had other options.

So, when I arrived back in Bondi after that year-long trip, I thought, 'I'm going to ease my way back into fitness'. I'd always been athletic and active through primary and high school. I was fiercely competitive, but that fire in my belly was extinguished by the depression. I wanted my edge back.

Admittedly, when I walked through the doors of the Dharma Shala in North Bondi (which back then, by the way, was the first yoga school in Bondi and ultra-traditional), I was nothing short of intimidated. Yoga was still considered 'new age' and 'herbal'. I had a pre-conceived idea that it was for girls (luckily, I was winning in that department) and for the spiritually elite (which I most certainly wasn't).

I rolled out the blue, sticky mat that I'm sure had seen many a sweaty session and sat down not knowing exactly what to do or expect. I looked around the room, trying not to seem like a complete novice, stared curiously at the carpeted floor and the deities on the wall and took in the occasional waft of burning incense.

I remember the moments leading up to class so vividly. There was a guy next to me lying down on his back, knees bent and soles of feet touching. He had his arms stretched above his head, eyes closed as if it were just him and his Darth Vader just-audible breath.

I was both charmed and nervous in this setting, but totally awake.

I fumbled my way through that first class (and many after) and felt like a baby elephant, stomping around the mat while everyone seemed to float, but by the end of class felt more at ease than I had in a while.

The state was unexplainable.

As I walked home from practice that night, I remember stopping in my tracks and standing still as if to honour something. It was the first time in a long time that I could 'feel' something. That word again.

And to feel was big for someone who had experienced neither the intensity of joy nor the sharpness of grief for a long while.

It was as though something had been stirred deep within and as I stood there silently, time ceased to exist. I could sense the temperature of my skin, the rhythm of my breath and a feeling of sadness for all the moments I'd missed these past few years. This was a really human moment: feeling the sadness and not suppressing it. Tears welled up and I felt a few escape.

'What is the yoga?' I wondered. Perhaps all that moving and breathing had touched parts of my body and lungs that previously had never been explored. I didn't know. But I was willing to try again. And I did.

Before I knew it, I was practising four to five times a week. My body changed in just a month. I felt stronger, leaner and way more alive. That was all a bonus, for the real gift for me (and every practitioner I know) was in the mind. I started to stress less about the small stuff at work, let things pass and focus on what really mattered.

My sleep improved, my digestive system (previously out of whack) was kicking and soon I came off my anti-depressants. I'd found a new coping mechanism. Yoga was, and still is, my medicine.

I was hooked. I would sit at my desk at lunch time and look up yogic philosophy, read interesting facts and look forward to my next dose.

I was working in advertising, with an incredible team who were supportive of my new addiction, and I just loved them to bits. We were like family. And with my own in the country four hours away, this was really important to me. But I knew the job itself wasn't right for me. You see, that's another side effect of practising yoga, the 'get really clear'.

At some point, holding onto what doesn't feel right becomes way more painful than flowering into what you know you can be.

I knew, incredibly early on in my yoga journey, that it would be a part of my life moving forward, but didn't have the confidence to voice it.

After a year and a half of yoga, another vivid and colourful, time-stand-still moment occurred. I'd finished a class one morning at the Shala (where I continued to loyally practise) and my teacher, Rick, stopped me on the way out and said, 'I think you'd make a really good teacher, Katie. You should think about doing your teacher training.'

Hair stood up on my skin. Every cell in my body was alert. Every part of me was ecstatic.

I looked up to Rick, and still do. He gave me the real deal experience in those early years and whenever I think of him, I still feel incredibly honoured and lucky. I haven't come across many like him since.

I learnt two things in that moment: yoga was going to be my life's devotion; and when you believe in someone, tell them.

That moment changed the direction of my life forever.

That day, on my lunch break, I started researching yoga teacher training and within six months I was on a plane to India, scared and excited and ready for this new chapter of my life.

Mumbai was a loud, bustling, altogether strange place for this country girl at heart. Yes, I'd spent half my life in Sydney after growing up in Batlow, a small town in southern New South Wales, but I was still rooted in the 'quiet' and felt more secure in stillness and calm than in noise and calamity. This was next level. And something strange happened in that overnight stay in Mumbai before I travelled south to Goa, where my training was to take place for the next two months. I got to the hotel room, locked the door and was paralysed with fear. I decided I didn't know if teaching yoga was right for me. Had I made the wrong decision?

Looking back, I learnt something else about myself: when fear creeps in, I doubt myself and back down. I retreat. I'm no longer 'all in'. The fear of failure can be too much to bear and my ego won't tolerate it. It doesn't mean I wasn't once fully committed, but for as long as fear takes centre stage, I'm half way out the door. And that's OK.

That aside, I loved the training and being in the quieter region of Goa – a place colonised by the Portuguese on the West Coast of India. I loved our weekend beach visits, complete with cows lazing around on the sand like they owned the place (well – they kind of do). I loved our Ayurvedic chef who made incredible meals and gave us specialised potions when we felt sick. She was an angel. Everything about India was magic. When my two months was up, though, I was ready to come home and find a job back in the safety of the design and advertising industry that I'd been in for the four years since finishing university. After all, I'd have a steady income and I was in my comfort zone. Yoga, I'd decided, would continue to be a large part of my life but teaching was not for me.

Now here's an example of just how wonderful and crazy and seemingly disorganised, yet so organised at the same time, life can be.

When I returned from India, we were feeling some of the side effects of the 2008 global financial crisis in Sydney. I struggled to find work. I got the odd temping job but nothing solid. It seemed life was against me. I wasn't sure when my next pay check would arrive, and I felt uprooted and unsettled.

I finally settled for a position not dissimilar to the one I had known wasn't right for me before I left for India; fear was running the show, so I bowed down to comfort. The company itself was on top of its game worldwide, but I felt lost and not quite at home. Not in a 'I'm out of my comfort zone' kind of way but more in a 'I'm not one bit passionate about this' way.

Another lesson transpired in the second week of this job.

I was at a party with a friend who managed a gym and she asked how my training in India had been. 'Incredible,' I said. 'Life changing. But I only did it for fun. Not sure I want to teach.' She looked at me knowingly, like she'd been there before, and tilted her head in curiosity. 'Really? Because I want to introduce yoga at the gym. I have a pile of resumes on my desk from yoga teachers who are keen but if you want the job, it's yours.'

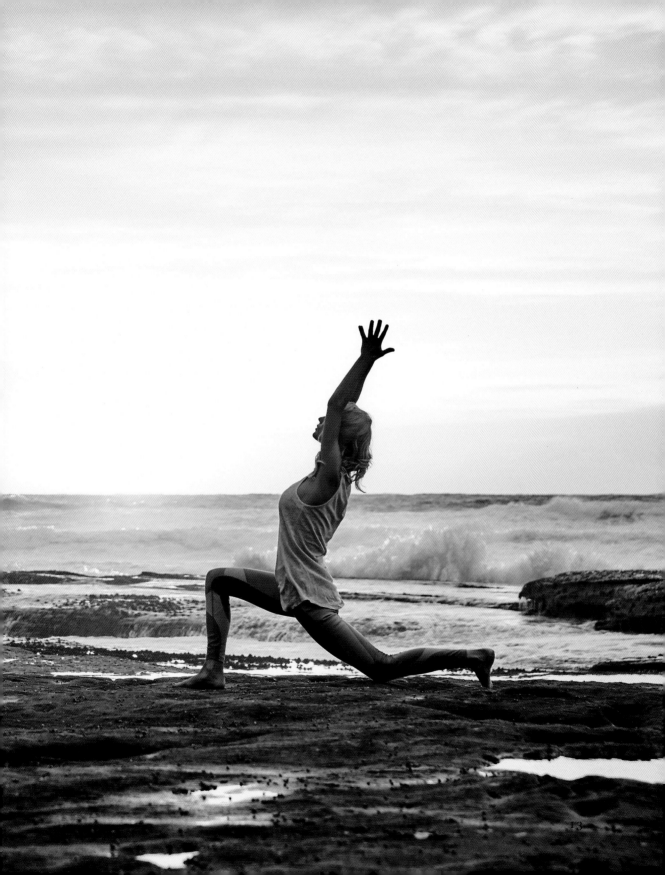

Boom. It was now or never. There are only so many times that opportunities like this come knocking on your door, before they start knocking on the door of the more courageous. I thought about it for a day and decided to take it. And that decision opened another door.

Another friend asked me to give him a month's worth of private lessons at his place twice a week, which then rolled on to be the next three years. And a good mate who worked for another gym asked me to lead some yoga classes for the South Sydney Rabbitohs rugby league team.

Doors just kept opening. And I now know that to be absolutely true of life.

When you're doing something you love, doors open and magic happens.

I spent the next two years teaching around Sydney's eastern suburbs and getting some pretty good gigs. I became an ambassador for fitness-wear brand Lululemon's Bondi Junction store. Lululemon were insanely good to me and are insanely good to so many fitness and yoga teachers worldwide. They taught me the importance of community (something that would go on

to be important to us at Flow Athletic), to support the human next to you and how to set goals for a rich and dreamy life.

During my time as an ambassador, I was invited to go to Whistler, Canada, for an ambassador summit where I would be joined by 100 other young yoga and fitness instructors from around the world. I was pinching myself. They were flying me to Canada and they were throwing tools at us for being entrepreneurs in the fitness industry. I had a ball and came back motivated to open my own studio, an idea that I'd been discussing with one of my clients for a few months prior to the trip.

Ben Lucas would come to my class religiously on Tuesday and Thursday afternoons at 4pm. He was pretty quiet.

One day he explained that he was training for an ultra-marathon and asked if I could give him private lessons twice a week. I said yes. And it was during these sessions that Flow Athletic was born.

He asked me why I didn't have my own studio. 'You have people lining up for your classes. You could really do it.' My response was the stock standard 'I don't have enough money, I'm not experienced enough and I don't know enough about business.'

To which he said, 'You'll never have enough money or experience or know enough. You just start.'

Wise advice.

Well, he's a wise human. And one of the best I've known. He'll always be the one who believed in me when I didn't. And that counts for a lot. I'm blessed, honoured and humbled to know him. He's a pillar of the community with a large heart and just wants to see people do well.

So it was upon returning from my trip to beautiful Whistler that I said to him: 'Right. I want to do this. But I want to do this with someone who knows what they're doing.' He had been in the fitness game for a long time and had three successful businesses, so it would be a big gamble for him to sell them all and create a business with me.

But he said yes. Although his businesses were thriving, he said there was no growing for him to do there and he didn't want to 'die with the music still in him'.

We started researching and deciding on our concept. We wanted it to be different and while I was giving him yoga lessons he started giving me personal training sessions. It really hit home that his sessions were strengthening my yoga practice and my yoga was making his recovery from training much quicker, plus he felt calmer and more energised.

It was a no brainer. We decided to combine the magic of yoga with fitness. Sure, you could go to a gym and do yoga, but at that stage in time it didn't feel like 'traditional' yoga. I was adamant that I didn't want to lose the tradition of magic in the process.

Flow Athletic opened March 18, 2013 and thanks to our unique concept, day spa fit-out, amazing branding (thanks Mervyn Tan!) and snappy PR we arrived with a bang. The first few weeks were relatively quiet – although we were never short of things to do – but then we got really busy.

And this is when things started to fall apart for me. Internally.

That first year of being in the business was amazing, golden and incredibly hard all at once. Any new business owner will tell you this. And with our business being a new model, Ben and I and the rest of the team spent all of those first few months in reaction mode.

There was always a fire of some sort to put out, a new challenge each day, and I felt way out of my depth. I knew there were times Ben felt so stressed that he wondered if he'd made the wrong decision.

And I was going through a hefty break up. I'd been engaged to be married and that was falling apart around the time we opened. It was the best and worst of times for that to happen: best because I was distracted by work and worst because I had moved out and was spending my evenings on friends' couches.

I stopped nourishing my body and taking my medicine – that is, practising yoga consistently. I set a frantic pace, never stopping to appreciate what we were building with Flow Athletic. I was always on my way somewhere and doing something, and although my body would be present when talking to someone, my mind would be racing on to the next 'to-do'.

I forgot how to savour the small things, such as a glass of wine with friends, a slow-cooked meal at home or taking myself off to a long, luxurious yoga class.

My friends would comment on how little I'd see them and how, when I did, I appeared scattered and 'not there'. I wasn't present. One friend actually referred to me as a zombie. That hit home.

This was in contrast to when I was at work, where I made myself 'switch on'. I felt like I had to uphold this reputation I had as the 'perfect' yoga teacher who had it all together. I hated displeasing people and saying no. The yoga community as well as our Flow Athletic community saw me as this fresh and vibrant yoga teacher who taught wellbeing and mindfulness for a living, but inside I was decaying and had been diagnosed with adrenal fatigue and burnout. I felt like a fraud.

Enough was enough. I took myself home to the country over Christmas and reminded myself what it was about yoga that I loved. The philosophy, the way it made me feel grounded and 'at home' in my body, and how it helped me slow down.

I started using some tools and philosophies that I'd learnt in yoga and mindfulness and made them a daily ritual. And the simplicity of them was pure magic. They worked. And I still use them today to slow down, reprioritise and 'come home'.

All of these tools cultivate an environment for 'living in flow'.

All of them, and more, are in this book.

Living in flow reminds me to choose dates with mates who give me belly laughs over deadlines that don't mean much; to be fierce but flexible in my pursuit of my goals;

and that the greatest gift we can give to others is connection and presence.

Living in flow means that you (the always on-the-go, busy, stretched in a million different directions kind of person) can reap the benefits of slowing down, savouring experiences and creating more meaningful connections. After all, I believe that's why we're here. Connection. And it's why there's a whole chapter dedicated to it in this book.

And when we live in flow for long enough, we observe the world around us change. When we're respecting ourselves and others, we're vibrant and wide awake, the right people and relationships show up and doors open wide to opportunities that we might imagine only in our wildest of dreams.

Sure – things still happen to throw us out of alignment, but once we've tasted 'flow', the incentive to get back to that nurturing state is more than enough.

What is life if we're merely existing and skimming over experiences? Let's live, dive deep and be curious of the world around us.

Let's live in flow.

How to use this book

I wanted this book to be both beautiful and truly useful.

As such, I recommend reading *Life in Flow* in its entirety. Choose a chapter a week, repeating the Moving Meditation three to four times during the week and exploring the concepts and philosophies of the chapter, then move on to the next chapter.

After completing the book, let the universal life force or flow do its magic. Pick up the book any time you feel the urge and randomly choose a page. No doubt something will 'hit' you in just the right way on that exact day. Or choose the Moving Meditation that appeals most to your mood at that time.

Sip. Savour. Slow down and thoroughly enjoy.

CHAPTER 1

Grounding

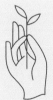

the art of slow

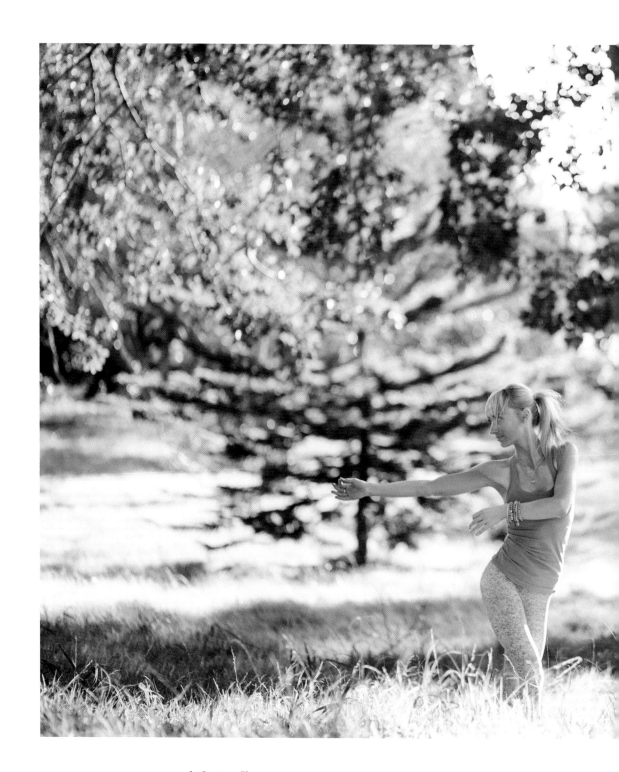

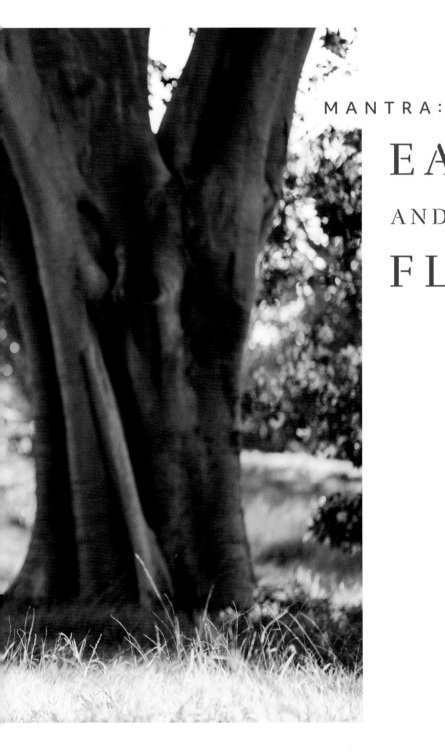

MANTRA:

EASE

AND

FLOW

"Nature does not hurry, yet everything is accomplished."

Lao Tzu, ancient Chinese philosopher

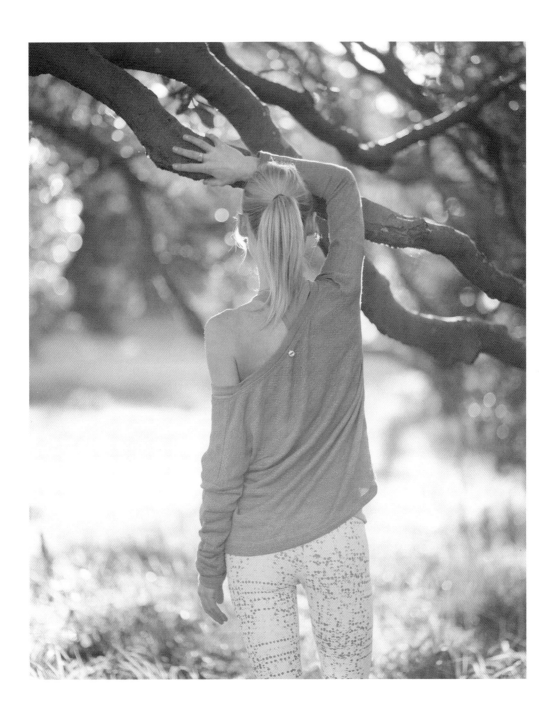

Grounded. It's a term used often by yoga teachers and meditation teachers alike. And... it can sound downright clichéd and trite when over-used and under-explained.

So what is it? And why is grounding so integral to our health, productivity and fulfilment?

In the simplest of terms, it's a felt sense of slowing down and being 'in your body', or inhabiting the whole space that is your physical body. It teaches us to savour the moment and live it fully. And when we live at this pace and in that state, we're less reactive, more clear-headed, calm and creative.

We suffer less and we live in wonder way more.

Grounding is a process of dynamic contact with the Earth. With so much spiritual emphasis on energy 'rising' and transcending the body, there should be just as much emphasis on energy in a downward direction, for it allows us to remember that we are solidly here in the now. When we connect with the Earth we sense its boundaries and edges, and although this may sound limiting, it creates a sense of security.

We all have those favourite things, right? A chair, a meal, surroundings. The things that help make us feel 'at home'. They help us feel rooted and like *us*. Without these things we feel unstable and off-balance. When we lose our ground, our attention wanders from the present moment. We are no longer 'in our body'.

Being grounded has the capacity to soothe and, often, to free us from stress and anxiety. It's the foundation for any mindfulness or meditation practice and perhaps one of the most under-trained skills we have in modern society.

It cultivates presence – and that is the essence of yoga. I think our children should be learning how to ground in school. I have a hunch it would deeply affect the globe's future.

Yep. I think fairly highly of grounding. It's a daily ritual for me. A game changer and an essential way to connect not only to myself, but also to nature and those around me. It's everything.

You see, in our busy day-to-day lives, we leave the body many times. And when I say 'leave the body', I mean we journey into the mind, which transports us out of the body into all kinds of illusions.

If you really observe, you'll notice that you're in your mind most of the time, from the moment you wake up.

The mind – although seemingly a part of your body – has the ability (and when applied mindfully, I say a 'super ability') to transport you. It can pour your awareness into all kinds of concerns and curiosities: adventures and events from the past and the 'what if' faraway places of tomorrow. Pretty neat. The problem is that you're likely sending your mind away from your home base (the body) too frequently, to the point where it can feel like you're uprooted, and immersed in thoughts that – when you really observe them – can be harmful.

If our thoughts create our reality, which is a common spiritual belief, then what we pour our mind into matters.

Grounding brings us back home to the body. More than this, it slows us down.

There are many pathways to 'coming home' that will be explored in this chapter, including awareness of the Earth underneath, awareness of breath and awareness of sensations, but only those with a secret super power can enter these paths: Slow.

Why we rush

I feel that now, more than ever, we're all pulled to, or curious about, grounding. And it's absolutely no coincidence that you've been pulled to or given this book.

We live life at a frantic pace. Sometimes it feels hard, impossible even, to jump off this speeding train ride we're on. And without a doubt, there are those of us who are addicted to busy.

Never have we had access to so many things, right now. We seem to have little tolerance for slow: slow services, slow transport, slow communication. The one thing we do seem to love is slow food (hallelujah) but even then... we kind of want it now so we get other people to make it for us, so that all we have to do is walk in, order and then boom. Slow on a plate. We've missed the point.

 Self Enquiry: When was the last time you left plenty of time in the morning to have a conscious conversation with a neighbour, or took the time to stop and listen to how a colleague or friend really is?

Since when did 'how are you?' become a passing comment like 'hi' and 'goodbye'?

Guilty as charged. The days when I'm most busy I get frustrated when someone wants to have a conversation. And why? When I pull myself out of the trance and remember what's most important, I lean in to the possibility that this person may just want to be heard. They may even have an answer to some of the questions I'm so frantically pursuing.

We all deserve to be heard and we all deserve connection. There's a philosophy that every person is put in front of us to teach us something. Every single person. Especially the people who press all our buttons the most. Imagine that.

Yogi 1

ANDREW KINGSTON
(AKA 'KINGO')

My mate and yoga student, Andrew Kingston, is just an ordinary guy – ordinary and extraordinary. He started coming to my classes when we opened Flow Athletic and soon became known and adored by our team as 'The Gift' because of his charm and good looks.

But behind the looks lies a soul that is insanely true and kind. And when someone asks me what a yogi is, it's him. A yogi, to me, may have never participated in a yoga class, nor know what downward-facing dog is, but they understand and practise 'presence'. That's a yogi.

When you speak with Kingo, it's as if it is just you and him in the room. He's never distracted by anyone or anything over your shoulder and he takes the time to ask you how you are and what you've been up to – and not only that, you can tell he's interested in your response.

I remember one morning when he'd finished a class. After showering and getting ready for work at a leisurely pace, while his fellow Flow athletes rushed and scampered for buses, he took breakfast out of his locker, sat in the community area and proceeded to slowly eat. It was such a good lesson for me. Slow down. Take time. Savour. It sets the tone for the rest of the day.

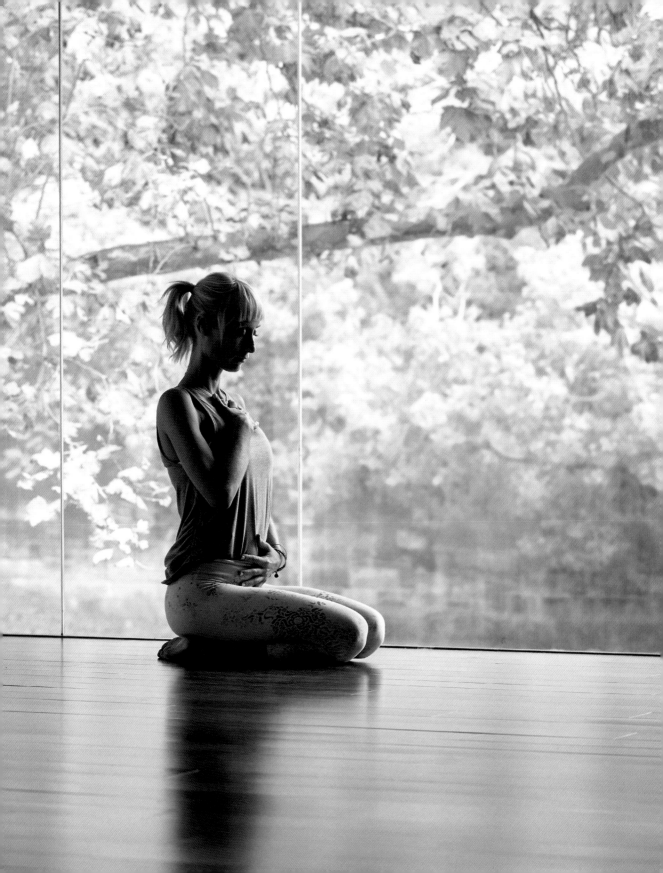

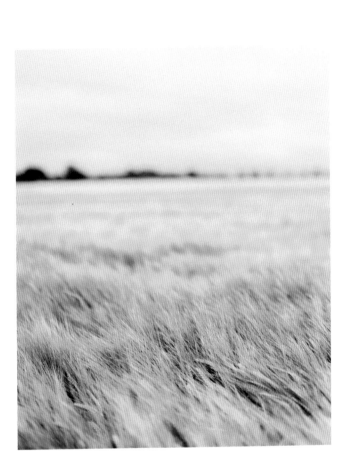

Slow is sexy

Kissing. Food.

Two things that can be super sexy when slow.

Dressing. Undressing. Dancing.

There's another three.

Personally, I find people who move through life at a calm pace, unaffected by the hectic world around them and focused on operating at their own speed, totally sexy. Man or woman. There's something magnetic about their ability to anchor to the moment and move through it with ease.

OK. Lean in and get real close – do any of the below resonate with you?

Do you, from the moment you wake to the moment you go to bed, fill your days with 'things to do'?

Is there always a voice inside your head telling you to do more, be more and achieve more?

Do you incessantly rush from one meeting, catch up or task to the next, leaving very little time for stillness?

Do you always feel rushed? Do you often feel as if you're rushing others? Do you get frustrated when others don't work at your pace?

Are you often late for things or pressed to make an appointment in time?

Do you sometimes hop in your car or jump on public transport and realise that when you arrive at your destination you can't even remember getting there?

Do you get to the end of your day and feel as if you've been pulled in every different direction doing things for others, yet you've accomplished nothing for yourself?

If you answered yes to any of the above, you could probably (like me) do with a good dose of slow to kickstart your dedication to grounding. Most of us not only repeat the same old thoughts and narratives internally each day, but also spend a good chunk of our time in a fast-paced, frenetic, reactive mode.

Reactive mode is rampant with rush, and ripe with regret.

You can get so busy fulfilling the needs of others that you habitually take on too much while your own dreams fade and wilt.

Here's what happens when you choose to slow down.

Your thoughts become more organised, prioritised and clear.

Your focus and quality of work improve.

You remember what your values are and what activities are aligned to them.

You're a kinder, more compassionate person (including to your barista, who is doing their best to get all those orders out at once!).

You work from a place that is calmer and less frenetic, meaning you ultimately make better lifestyle choices, with clarity and groundedness.

You become the kind of person that you want to hang out with.

own
the
flow

SLOW DOWN

For one week, slow everything down.

Make a conscious effort to eat slower, talk slower, 'make-out' slower, work at a slower pace. Take time in the morning to get ready without rushing out the door and create space between your 'to dos' and chores to let things process.

When you're showering, take your time. When you're preparing meals, slow down. And when you're feeling that incessant need to push faster, go harder and force something, yes, that's your cue to SLOW DOWN.

The moments you feel like the world might end if you slow down? That's when you need to slow down the most.

Sure – there are times to hustle and make things happen. There are times to push further, to go hard, to pull the all-nighter when you're on a critical deadline. But otherwise... slow down.

It sounds counter-productive but often the slower and more deliberate you are, the more you get done. And when we feel productive and like we're getting things done, we feel fulfilled. Only always.

Slowing down allows your cells to rejuvenate and restore so that in the times the hustle is really needed, you can go full throttle and kick goals.

Do you want to race to the end of your life? Or do you want to slow down, drink in your moments and savour the sweetness of what every moment has to offer?

Slow down. Let yourself catch up.

Tomorrow night, spend just five minutes journalling your 'slow' experience. Write down anything at all that you have observed, from frustration and resistance to joy and clarity.

Mindfulness is like a muscle: the more we practise it – in this case, being aware of pace – the stronger it becomes.

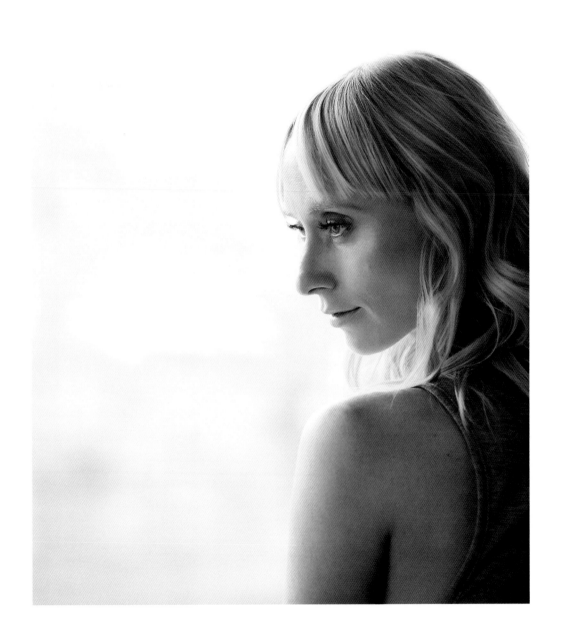

mantra | ease and flow

It's time to lean in, root down and surrender to the solid structure
below: earth. We can all have a rich and dynamic relationship
with it. Trust it. Feel it. Be it. Repeat the mantra to yourself
silently whenever your mind wanders.

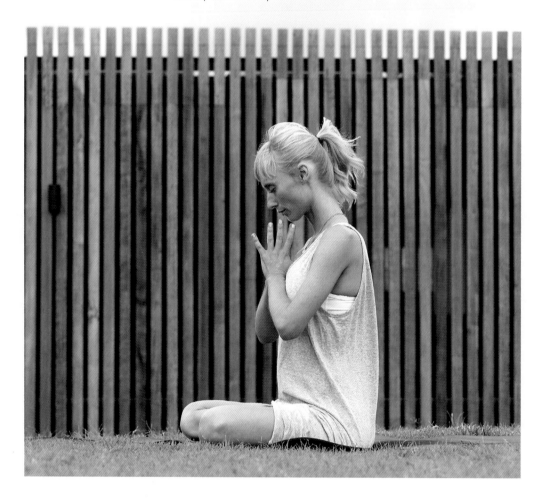

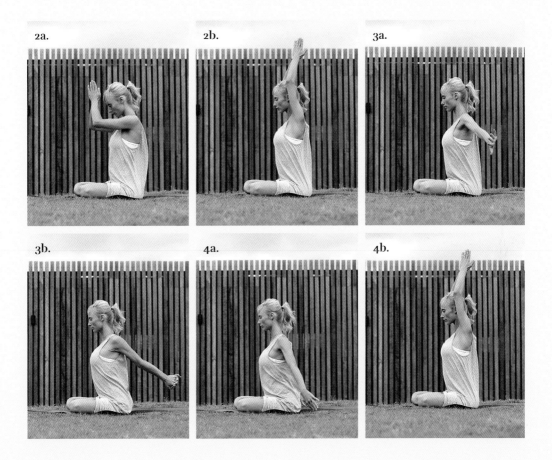

2a.   2b.   3a.   3b.   4a.   4b.

1 Cross-Legged Namaste Come into a cross-legged posture with hands at heart and chin gently into throat. Pause here for a few moments to ground and centre by closing your eyes and bringing your awareness to your base – your sit bones and the heavier bones of the legs. These are your anchor into this moment. At the same time there is an upward and outward motion into your spine, which feels awake yet at ease. If you are having trouble keeping the spine lifted, sit on a cushion or block. For your first round through steps 2–5 following on from here, spend five breaths in each stage. For the following rounds – do six in total – use one breath per movement.

2 Inhale and, keeping the hands together, lift your arms right up above the head.

3 Exhale, separate the hands and take your arms out to the side and back to interlace your hands behind you. Inhale and ease your knuckles down and back. Stay in the posture and breathe into the chest. Stay here for the exhalation.

4 Inhale. Arms move back up above head until palms touch.

5.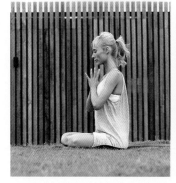

6a.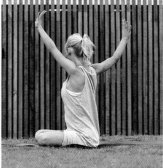

6b.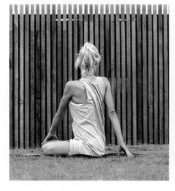

6c.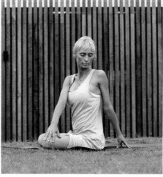

5 Exhale the hands down through the midline of the heart, returning to namaste or prayer position with the hands. Repeat the above sequence five times and then finish with the following.

6 Seated Twist After the rounds of steps 2–5, inhale the arms out to the side and up to lengthen the spine and then exhale to twist to the right, placing the left hand to the right knee and the right hand behind you. Take an inhalation to lengthen the spine and an exhalation to gently twist to the right. Inhale the arms up above head. Exhale, twist to the left side and repeat.

7 Cross-Legged Forward Fold Take the right shin in front of the left with heels away from sit bones to form an upside-down triangle. Keep feet active to protect the knees. Inhale the arms above the head, interlace the hands and tilt forward from the hips as you exhale. Keep the spine long. Inhale to slowly come up. Switch legs and repeat, returning to cross-legged namaste to flow through the sequence as many times as feels good.

Remember: ease and flow. Take this with you off the mat and into the day.

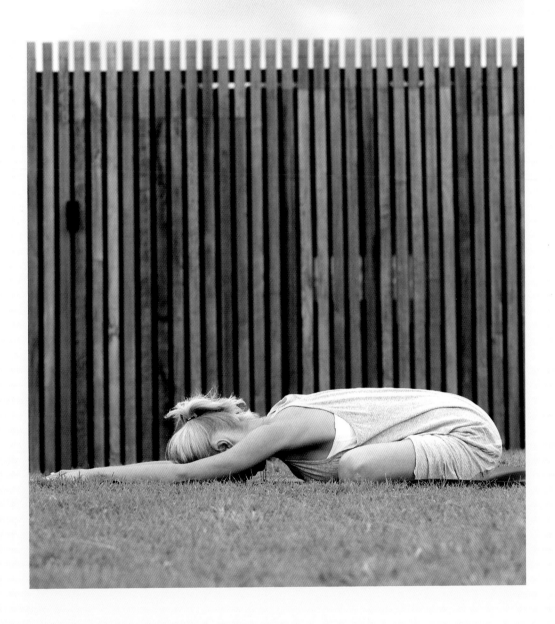

7.

The pathways to 'grounded'

I've picked up a few neat tricks on my yoga journey that have helped me slow, settle and ground.

God knows I've needed them. Indeed, I don't know how people cope without grounding or some kind of ritual.

There's no one size fits all; some grounding techniques may work well for you, while others may not. Part of your path is finding what suits you.

From teachers, retreats, my own teaching experience and exploration, here are my favourites.

Try some on. See what fits.

Make friends with the Earth

When I teach yoga, I like to keep it playful and fairly sensory driven. If I apply visuals they're taught as an exploration of the internal scenery. Everything I teach is designed to keep you at home and in your body.

One such sensory experience is to connect with, or make friends with, the Earth. If we are mindful of the support and sensation of what's underfoot, we're immediately drawn to the lower part of the body – which yoga says is the best place to ground or re-root.

Think of your body as a tree. When you feel wobbly and ungrounded, distracted and vague, you can feel like you're 'uprooted', right? I know

I can. I feel like I've lost my footing or lost my way. Grounding through the feet and acknowledging your connection to the Earth re-roots, re-plants and deeply connects you to the moment.

Grounding in this way has other benefits. When we feel a connection to the Earth, we connect to something larger than ourselves, which reminds us of our connection to all things and beings. And this is largely the basis of our yoga practice.

Connection – it's why we're here.

And when we remember our connection to the Earth – the planet all humans are a part of – it can make our big issues seem small in perspective.

In energy anatomy (a really cool subject that you learn when studying yoga), it's believed that various sites on the physical body relate to different aspects of our lives and psyche. And when those energy sites are 'out' or misaligned, it can have an impact on our health. This is talked about in the chakra system.

When we feel uprooted, we can experience health issues, our finances may be out of whack, our home can be messy, there may be family conflict. There is likely to be a disruption to our sense of community and connection to others (this is looked at in Chapters 3 and 4). But the great thing about this is that we always have a choice and we can use the practices of yoga to become more aligned. More on this later.

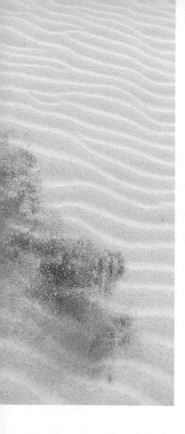

own
the
flow

INTO THE EARTH

Wherever you are right now, take a moment to be still. Close your eyes and let your awareness fall to the soles of your feet. Feel all four corners of your feet firmly press down into the Earth as if you're sinking a few centimetres below. As you press down, feel it press back up in support. Take three or four easy breaths.

The philosophy that ties in with this simple action is this: *Our bodies – the microcosm of the macrocosm.* There's an ancient yogic philosophy that our bodies are just miniature versions of the universe. It states that what we do to ourselves, we do to others. And it's why grounding and, in particular, re-connecting with the Earth and nature, reminds us to be kind to the environment.

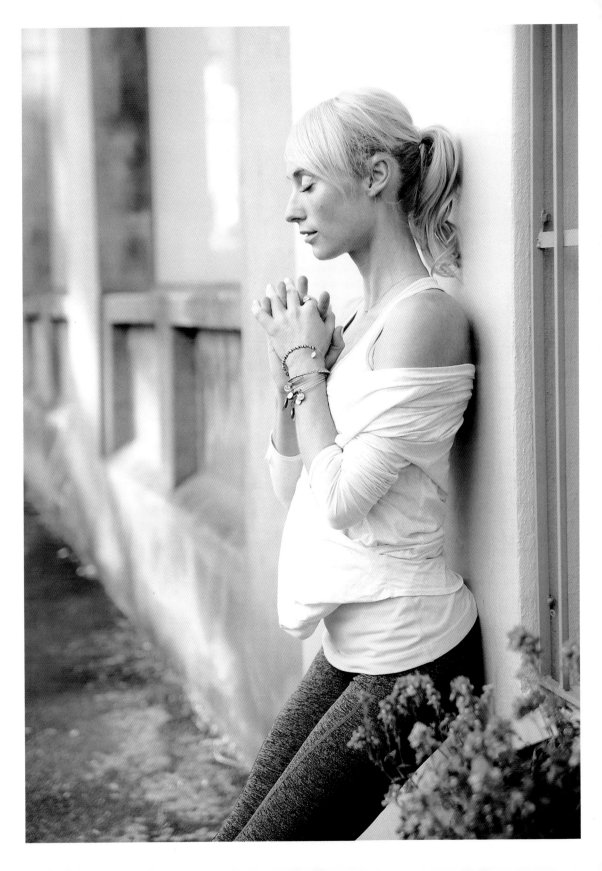

Move your body

When was the last time you trained, practised yoga or went on a brisk walk and regretted it? Often the times when we're feeling the most scattered, vague or disconnected are the moments we most need to move the body. All that messy energy needs to go somewhere, right?

From the moment I took my first class, yoga has been my medicine and still is. Almost daily. Aside from Sunday when I lay pretty low, most days I practise for anywhere between 15 and 90 minutes. A combination of conscious breathing, strength work and dynamic movements, sealed with calming forward bends, brings me back into my body and leaves me profoundly grounded.

Running and strength sessions are other ways to move towards groundedness for me. There's nothing like that feeling of applying so much effort that afterwards you feel totally vibrant, lit up and alive. It's also a really good example of how being grounded doesn't necessarily have to mean you're totally calm and mellow.

You can be grounded while delivering a pitch alive with energy for work, playing a game of hockey or even just driving your car. As long as you're 'in your body', you're grounded.

If you're feeling 'uprooted' from some kind of trauma, such as the death of someone close, an accident, or a heavy and confronting argument with a partner, I think one of the healthiest things you can do for yourself is move.

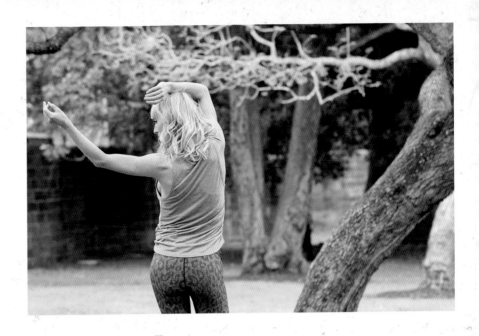

I remember being about eight years old and watching TV at my grandparents' house in Tumut, a neighbouring town to where I grew up. It must have been a *National Geographic* or nature show of some type because there was a bear who had almost been savaged by another. As the threatening bear left the scene, the traumatised bear began to shake. And shake and shake and shake until it seemed he had shaken the trauma out of his body. Finally, his breath deepened; he appeared to be relaxed and headed off, it seemed, to go about his day as usual.

I've seen birds do it when they slam into a glass door. At first, they lie still, seemingly dead. 'Poor birdie,' I always think, and then moments later the bird begins to shake until she also shakes it out completely, stands on her two little feet, fluffs up her wings and flies away.

Imagine if we dealt with trauma and emotions in the same way. Moment by moment, when things affect us, we could feel them and let them go instead of holding onto them and letting them fester inside the body for a lifetime. One of my top five favourite books, *The Untethered Soul* by Michael A. Singer, goes into this in great detail. Read it.

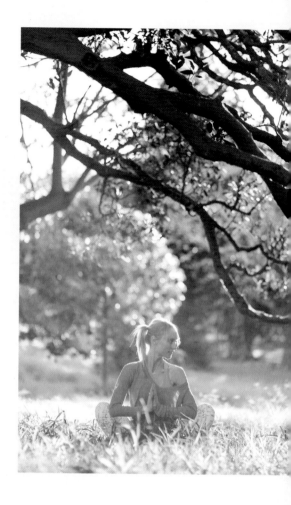

own
the
flow

MOVE AND RELEASE

Choose your medicine of choice: yoga
(I suggest vinyasa, ashtanga or power yoga
for this), dancing, running... any activity
in which you can be relatively physical.

Step 1. Acknowledge: Before you begin
the activity, acknowledge what it is that's
frustrating you, making you sad or
dragging you down. And if you can't work
out what it is, acknowledge the uncertainty.

Step 2. Dedication: Dedicate the activity
to releasing what you've acknowledged.

**Step 3. Shake it out through conscious
movements in the practice.** Do it. Feel it.

Step 4. Sacred Space. Take a moment
afterwards to notice how you feel. If
practising yoga, this would be done in
savasana. Check in with the 'aliveness'
of your body: the beat of your heart, the
temperature of your skin, the flickers
and pulses of sensation within. This is
your wildness. Feel it.

*Remember – being in your body and out
of your head is the whole point.*

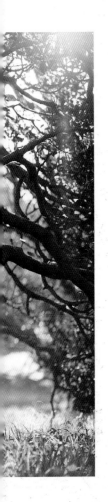

Date with nature

Spend an hour in nature and you'll feel the effects. Spend a week and you'll remember what it feels like to be in harmony with the living, breathing world around you.

So much time spent indoors and at a desk can have detrimental effects on our health. We know this. Yet so often we wait until we're on holidays or special occasions such as retreats to properly immerse ourselves in the great outdoors.

There's no specific Own the Flow for this one. Just get out there and breathe. Look at trees, listen to water falling or moving, watch the birds. Remember your connection to all of it.

There's a term, biophilia, which means 'love of life or living systems', and within the exploration of this delicious word is the healing power of nature.

There's a very special place in a very special part of the world that I visit. After a week there, I feel free and open wide.

Aro Hā is an adventure-wellness retreat just out of Queenstown on the South Island of New Zealand. In addition to being one of the most picturesque places I've laid eyes on, with majestic snow-capped mountains, glassy lakes and low hanging clouds (and this is just the view from the spa), there is an emphasis on getting back to your natural rhythms that makes it 'next level'.

I won't reveal the structure of the week as that's part of the mystery and charm of the experience, but I will say that there is a truly magic formula made up of nourishing food, no stimulants, space and time to reset and (the most important ingredient of all, I say) long stretches spent in nature. I think if we could all book in for a retreat like this every year, the world would be a more harmonious place.

Meditate

The game changer. Until around five years ago, the only meditation I really did was at the end of my asana practice. We'd finish a long, luxurious savasana, slowly make our way up into a seated posture and then sit, sipping in some further stillness and observing the inner environment. And this felt calming. Like it really 'sealed' the practice, you know?

Many may not know this but the original intention of the asanas (the physical postures in yoga) was to sit in meditation. That's all. Certain postures would be practised centuries ago so that yogis could sit for longer periods of time, more comfortable with open hips and a primed spine in meditation.

Somehow, here in the West, we've taken the practice and turned it into a multi-billion-dollar industry, quite often with the intention to create longer, leaner limbs and flat stomachs. All of this is a great side effect and a gift and total bonus to the practice, but that original intent was for stillness. Just to sit. And observe. And practise 'being'.

Fancy that.

About five years ago, my meditation practice went next level. And I still have so much to learn. I did a Vedic Meditation course run by my friend Jacqui Lewis of The Broad Place, a centre in Sydney that offers courses in integrated meditation to help bring creativity and consciousness into our daily lives. I went through a ritual to be 'inducted', learnt about the technique and then got sent out into the world to use it as a daily tool, twice a day.

In the Vedic style we 'sit' for 20 minutes each time. After the first few moments of settling into the seat (you don't have to sit cross legged in lotus – no way. You can sit on a chair and be comfy!), you begin

silently repeating the mantra that your teacher gives you during
that initial induction ceremony.

The mantra acts as a vehicle upon which the attention gently rests.
This allows the mind to settle into increasingly subtle levels of
thinking. Finally, the mantra transcends into a settled silence.

Oh and the mantra, you're told, is neither to be shared with others,
nor talked about. There is, I find, a certain mystery around it. And
I like that. Just like life. I don't need to know all the details but
rather feel the vibration. It's a meaningless sound so that we don't
go into the 'depths' or the context of the word – which only promotes
activity in the mind – and it has a vibration or resonance. This is said
to both attract and charm the mind.

The mantras used in this form of meditation and in yoga come from
the Vedic tradition of India and the Sanskrit language. It's said that
Sanskrit is the closest possible human imitation of the natural
vibrations produced from pure consciousness. Pure consciousness
is the source of all creation. It's how the unmanifest becomes the
manifest. And it's how the yogis believe the universe was created.

It's said that mantras have healing powers for specific parts of the
body, but the ones in the Vedic tradition are transcendental, meaning
that they are used to at first settle or ground us into the body and
then as we transcend we become aware that we're not just this body;
that we're very much connected to all of creation.

It's a lot to wrap your head around, huh? I know. I feel you.

But it's with a steady, patient and tender practice that we slowly
listen, feel and download the wisdom.

One conscious breath

This is my direct route to 'grounded'. And unless I'm in the middle of some deep trauma or catastrophe (in those times I need something a little more heavy duty), it works. Every time.

This one can be done anywhere and anytime. It's easy-peasy and something we do naturally all day, every day. It's just that 98 per cent of the time, we're unaware of the fact that we're doing it because we're lost in a trance of 'busy-ness'.

Breathing.

Most of the time we zip from one thing to another unaware that we're not breathing to our full potential. If stressed or anxious, we'll tend to breathe into the chest region, leading to shallower breaths and possibly exacerbating the state we're in.

If we learn to breath 'consciously' right down into the lower lobes of the lungs, we activate the parasympathetic nerve receptors, which chills us out and calms us right down[1].

One conscious breath will change your state. Immediately.

own
the
flow

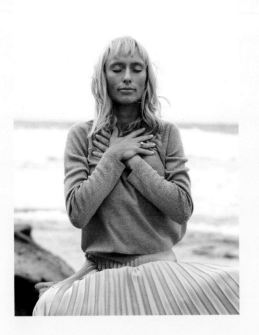

SLOW BREATH

Wherever you are, take a moment to either
softly gaze at a low point in front of you
or close your eyes. Take one hand to the
abdomen and the other just above. Take
a generous but gentle breath in, feeling
the hands lift and a long, slow breath out,
feeling the hands drop. Repeat as many
times as necessary.

Remind yourself: You are exactly where
you are meant to be. This isn't a mistake.
Take a deep breath and root yourself
in trust.

"Grounding is a daily ritual for me, an essential way to connect not only to myself but to nature and those around me. It's everything."

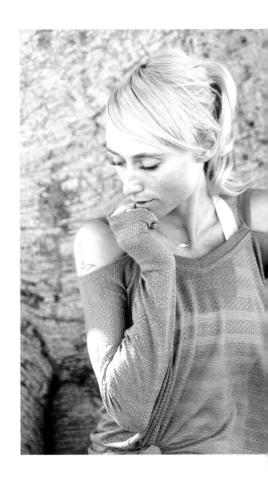

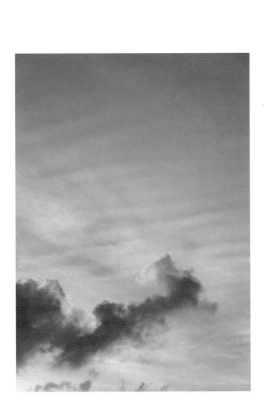

PHILOSOPHY 101.
The space between

I remember when I first started practising yoga. It was as if I was opening the door to some mystical kingdom.

There were so many 'aha' moments and rich philosophical concepts and learnings that were unheard of or unmentioned in my upbringing of Catholicism and country living. It was profound.

One such profound moment occurred when I was in paschimottanasana (a forward fold). Somehow my focus managed to sink down and away from the mind and into the depths of my breath. And in particular, into the space between my exhalation and inhalation, which is called bayu kumbhaka in Sanskrit.

It was in this space that, just for a few moments, my whole body was still as well as my mind (if only for a flicker). It felt like pure bliss; a moment of uninterrupted calm and clarity. And it was in this space that my body dropped physically deeper into the posture – a true testament to the notion that our mind holds tension and stores it in the muscles, ligaments and joints. When we free the mind, we free the body.

I went on to name, at first for myself as a reference point, this pure space between the breaths (which can also be experienced between the inhalation and the exhalation – antara kumbhaka) as The Space Between.

The notion of The Space Between grew, to become the place between thoughts; the space between mindless activities and the place where I felt most rested, at ease and expansive.

And then I began to extend the notion further.

What if The Space Between just became The Space and all of our activities were mind-FULL, filled with presence and the sensation of that pure place that I first experienced between breaths?

I have to remember, however, that we're human and part of our human experience is to be hijacked by fear and live out of The Space, in distraction or in flight mode. That's OK. But we can certainly try to live in The Space more often; to be more grounded, conscious and clear humans.

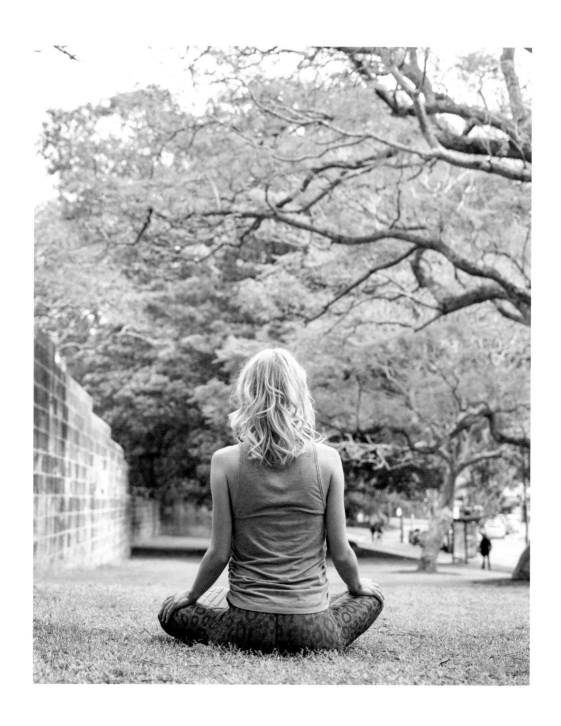

Grounding – the home base for creativity, clarity and change

Many yoga practices, such as Kundalini yoga, focus on liberating energy in an upward direction. However, this liberation must begin at the base, in what we call the root chakra or muladara chakra.

If you think about a tree, there's no way it's growing taller and more expansive if it's uprooted. It must be firmly planted, deep within the Earth, in order to grow.

In other words, you must first get totally grounded in the body before you can transcend it. Only then can you truly appreciate that you are not just this body; that you're capable of creating and manifesting big and wonderful things.

I mentioned in the introduction to this book my relationship to Lululemon, the Canadian-born athleisure-wear business. I did a short stint of working on the floor in the business while I was gathering up enough yoga clients and classes to sustain it as a full-time gig. During the first week of working for the showroom in Bondi Junction, I was taken for lunch with the store manager and asked what my goals were. What was my vision.

These were big questions for someone who didn't plan any further than lunch time.

A funny thing happens when you get real about what you really want.

I sat down and wrote out one-year, five-year and 10-year goals. I got excited. Life was going to be mammoth for this kid from the country.

And then it came time to verbalise these goals and read them out to my store manager. I got shy. I second guessed myself and wondered if I was worthy of all that I dreamed of.

Something magic happens when you write down goals and visions. They actually come to fruition.

Here's the process with making shit happen.

 You have an idea. You visualise it. You voice it. You connect with it so that it's heart felt. You may even get other people on board, people who share the same heart connection to it. You get disciplined about it. You find creative ways to make it happen. And boom... you hold it in your hand. It becomes form.

Through this process, I learnt something else.

You've got to be clear and careful about what you ask for. Because, if you follow the process, the universe almost always delivers.

I learnt that sometimes I set goals to please others or because I liked the idea of achieving them (ego based).

Have you ever set a goal, worked towards it and ticked it off, only to find that you felt nothing?

Shortly after opening Flow Athletic, one of my dear students, Ozlem, approached me after class and handed me a pink, purple and orange book called *The Desire Map*, by Danielle LaPorte. She said, 'I hear you talk in class, love your language and just think you'd enjoy this book.' I was due to go out that night so I sat down intending only to read a few pages over a cuppa and before I knew it, it was midnight and I had read the entire book. I was mesmerised and totally invigorated with this new philosophy on goal setting.

I recommend reading it but, in a nutshell, LaPorte stresses the importance of not just setting goals but getting clear on how you want to FEEL. She offered a solution to that 'meh-ness' I felt when I hit a milestone that I had thought I really wanted to hit. It's because I was working towards the goal out of obligation, instead of choosing how I wanted to 'feel' every day.

She suggests getting clear on your core desired feelings and set goals based around them. It worked a treat and when I grounded myself in a ritual each morning with the intention of cultivating those feelings, I attracted them. If one of my core desired feelings was 'nourished', for example, everything I did that day, every project I chose for the coming weeks, every person I chose to hang out with, would be in some way aligned to nourishing me. Mentally, physically and emotionally.

Being grounded and totally clear in a core desired feeling meant that I could decide really quickly if running a marathon was going to make me feel 'golden'. Or if opening another yoga studio would make me feel 'joyous'. Get my drift?

Pure magic. Thanks Danielle.

The golden rule – get grounded, be clear on how you want to feel and from that place of alignment, follow the process and make it happen. If you become misaligned, just have the discipline to get back on track.

Discipline creates a whole lot of freedom.

And remember the golden rule – if nothing else – SLOW DOWN.

Joy riding

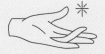

remembering what makes you happy

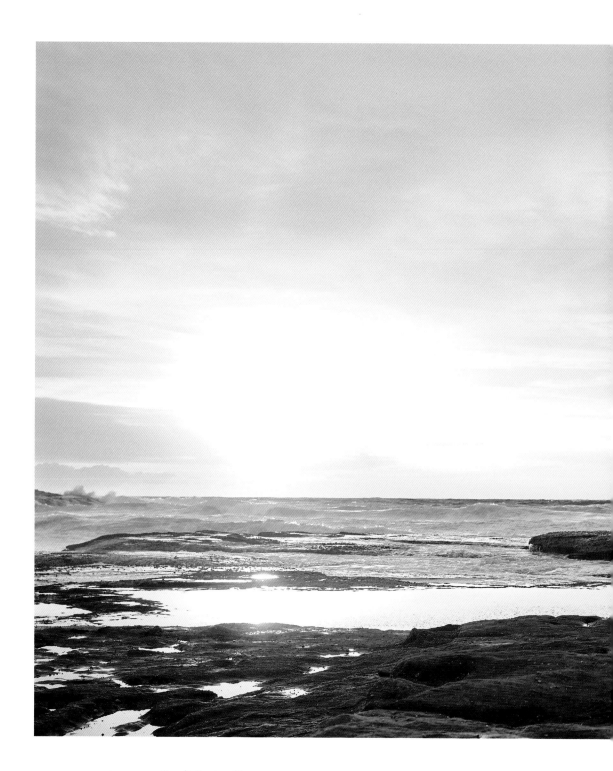

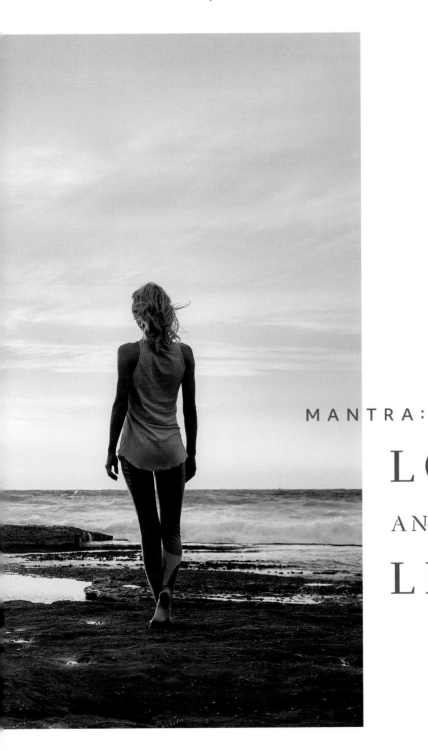

MANTRA:

LOVE

AND

LIGHT

"The most wasted of all days is one without laughter."

Nicolas Chamfort,
French writer, 1741–1794

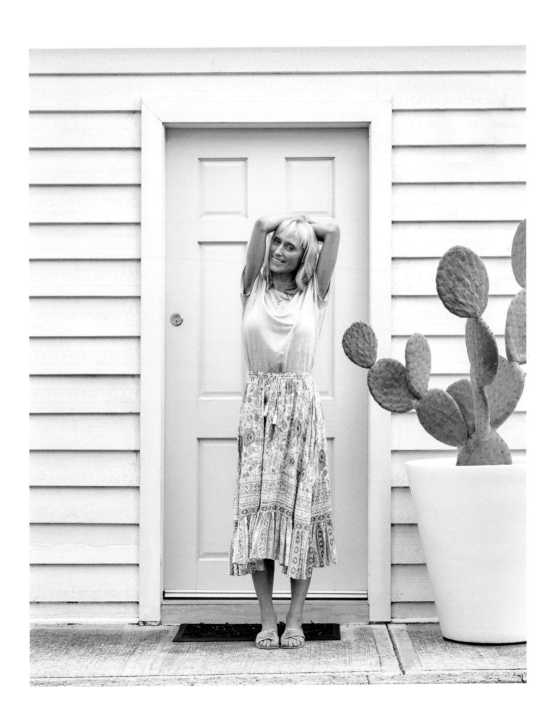

A few years ago, just after my burnout – I guess you could call it recovery time – I went on the first trip (of many) to a very sacred place called Aro Hā on the South Island of New Zealand. I call it sacred because it's somewhere I feel expansive, open and so deeply connected to myself and nature.

And there's a reason why. I talked about biophilia briefly in the previous chapter and how being out among nature has the capacity to heal and to bring you back to your natural rhythms. On this retreat we spend around three hours a day hiking on the most spectacular NZ trails. You're right in the thick of it and completely immersed.

Then there are the spa rituals, the clean, plant-based food and so many other things that go together to concoct just the right recipe for a soul-expanding experience like none other. It truly is remarkable.

On this particular retreat, near the end as all the 'ingredients' begin to sink in, we had a session called Peace Sticks. Part of the charm of Aro Hā is the mystery surrounding it – the unknown – so I don't want to expose every one of its secrets, but I will say that at the beginning of this session we're asked to reveal our 'Spirit Animals', which is all in good fun. Because that's actually the whole point of Peace Sticks: to have fun. To let go. To play. By the end of this session, having worked up a sweat, learnt a new skill and 'played' in a way I hadn't in a long time (perhaps since I was a kid) I began to cry.

The best kind of tears. Tears of joy; heart-felt, heart-opening and completely freeing tears.

It was totally liberating and I walked away from that session with the lightness of a child who knows no responsibility, and bears no guilt, shame or fear.

Do you remember that feeling?

Joy was the very secret ingredient to that feeling of expansion and lightness.

But why has it become such a secret?

Perhaps it's because we try so hard to find it when really, it's always there. Maybe we just cover it up.

The Buddhists would say so. They believe that joy is our nature and they simply call it 'Buddha Nature'. They believe that we are born this way.

And I believe it to be so. I believe we're all born joyous but somewhere along the path of development, amid external influences and the general baggage we decide to pick up and carry as our own, it gets suppressed, sometimes never retrieved, but often found in the unlikeliest of places.

A belly laugh with a good friend.

The savouring of a fine glass of shiraz on a cold evening by the fire.

In the eyes of a newborn.

Doing what you were born to do.

In the giving of a gift.

In a good book that touches your heart in just the right way.

During a yoga class.

Running as the sun rises.

Joy is everywhere. And there are two ways in which it happens. Let's look at this a little later on in this chapter. For now, believe that it's right there inside of you and just wants to bust open.

Re-prioritising joy

and why we lose touch with it in the first place

I remember as a kid jumping on my bike and playing for hours up and down the dusty country roads with my neighbour. We'd roam around the property I grew up on as a kid in Batlow (a small country town, famous for apples, in southern New South Wales).

We'd explore, adventure, build jumps, crash our bikes, speed through the orchards and generally run amok.

Five or six hours would pass before I'd even think about the time.

It's something kids do well – being present in the now and exploring what the moment has to offer. All done with pure bliss and curiosity.

I didn't know it back then because I was too consumed with being a kid, but that was living in the present moment – pouring my whole heart into the then and there.

And that, my yogi friend, is the foundation of mindfulness.

Soon enough, things changed. I grew up, added different dimensions to my personality (a result of peer influences), experienced fear, took on society's perceptions of what 'should' be and changed my playful attitude into one of seriousness and goal-orientated living. This is all a part of growing up. It's natural.

But what's not so natural is the giving up on joy part. That's something that should be kept and cherished.

It wasn't until one day five years ago that my mum said I was getting 'elevens' (apparently this is the name for the two lines you make in between the eyebrows when frowning and that everyone these days is getting Botox for) and to stop stressing. She'd caught me deep in a serious thought about something that felt very heavy and dark.

For the sake of looking good, I decided (yes – out of vanity – but hey – whatever gets you to that point, right?) to stress less. But, like anything, it takes practice. How good would it be to tell yourself, 'OK, today marks the day I don't stress any more.' And like magic. Whoosh. It's gone. Well, ultimately this can happen, but for most of us mere mortals it takes daily rituals, discipline and a few really stressful moments in which to truly test your new yogi superpowers against stress. It means:

Prioritising joy.

Carving space in our weekly schedule to dip into the things that cultivate joy.

Hanging out with friends who make us laugh and see the lighter side of life and being that friend for others.

It's the small things that really make a difference.

Have you ever noticed that the things that really bring joy to your life get put on the back burner and replaced by work and obligations?

Well. What if today were the day we started to re-prioritise for real?

You know that cheesy old line that asks, 'How would you live today if it were your last?' Have you actually stopped to think about it? What would you do? I like to extend it out to a week because it selfishly gives me more time to do more of the things that bring me joy. And when I tally up those things, there's a lot.

When I first did this exercise, I was astounded at what I was missing out on. 'Am I kidding?' I thought. 'Whose life am I living, anyway?'

There's something in everybody that waits and listens until you're completely open and in a 'whole-body-yes' state. It's the only true guide you'll ever have to following your dreams, making a real difference in this world and creating meaningful connections. And if you don't make space to set it free, you'll spend your whole life living by other people's rules.

That thing is joy.

Joy is an indicator that you're on the right track, that you're listening to your heart and that you're living your truth.

To get to joy, however, sometimes you have to feel the sharpness of pain. That's just a universal truth and often, though not always, the way through. It's part of being 'whole'.

Watch your world change when you re-prioritise joy.

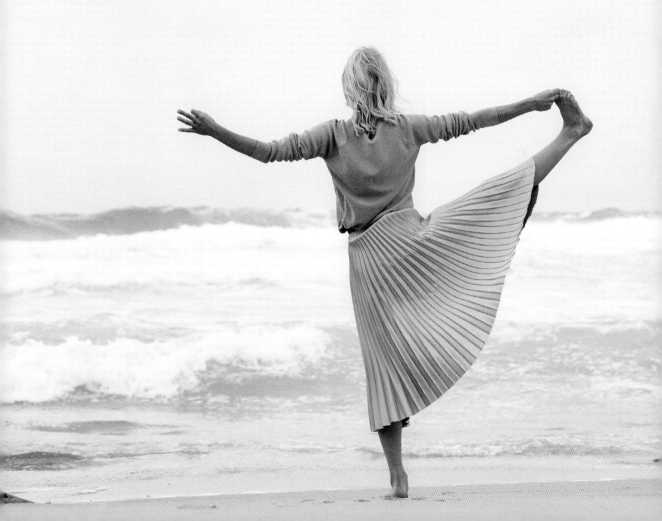

"Joy, it's been inside us all along."

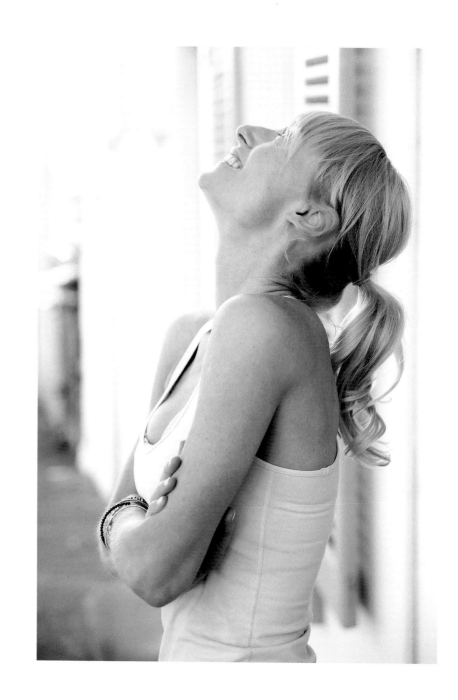

own
the
flow

WHAT MAKES YOU HAPPY?

So.

What makes YOU happy?

It's time to get clear.

Declare it to the world or just your journal. However you express it – get clear. Knowing what makes you happy could be the difference between living a life of 'meh' and 'hell yeah!'. And I think we all want 'hell yeah!'. So own it. Sit down, light a candle, make a cuppa or pour a glass of wine and put pen to paper.

What makes you happy?

The next step is to clear space in your calendar to do these things. Don't wait for the right time. Pick three of those things to do this week, another three the week after (some might be repeated) and then the same for the following two weeks. And before you know it, you have a month of joy planned. Make them non-negotiables.

Here are some of mine.

A beer with my mate Macca who gives me the biggest belly laughs of all.

Curling up on the couch on a rainy day with a good book.

Catch-ups with the girls.

Yoga class.

Nature hangs.

Spending time with my partner.

Adventures with my mum (even if it's just a coastal walk, or as far as trekking in Peru).

Spending time on my own, to recharge.

Writing.

Going to the movies and eating popcorn.

Listening to 'KK's Faves' playlist (a selection of my current favourite songs on Spotify).

Making soup.

"Life is a series of natural and spontaneous changes. Don't resist them – that only creates sorrow. Let reality be reality. Let things flow naturally forward in whatever way they like."

Lao Tzu, ancient Chinese philosopher

Impermanence

The river of change

Life is changing not just every once in a while, but always. This is one of the biggest universal truths, yet perhaps one of the hardest for us to embrace.

Every living thing, project, place and relationship has a life cycle; a beginning, middle and end. And as morbid as some endings may seem, really it just paves the way for a new beginning; a new creation; new life.

In hindsight, when we look back at the endings of a lot of things, we can see there was a 'why'. It was as if the universe had a grand plan for you that you just couldn't see at the time. Remember that relationship that came to a heart-breaking end and you thought you'd never get over it? And now, three years on you knew the gods were on your side because you fell into an even deeper love with someone else?

Yep. The only thing that is truly certain in this world is change.

Did you know that your body is replacing its cells with new ones at millions per moment?

The job that you're in right now will most likely change; you'll get a promotion or move on to start something new.

The nature of the relationship you're in right now may change. Perhaps it will deepen and then shallow. There may be children who alter the flow of your relationship, and when they grow up and you retire, the nature of your relationship will change again.

Mother Nature – one of our greatest teachers of all if we just listen to her – is forever orchestrating change. We feel and see change in her change all year round.

We know change to be a fact of life. And often we embrace it.

At the end of summer, I'm always so excited at the opportunity to don my UGG boots and dressing gown, and when winter ends I'm pumped to get back onto my tank tops and tiny shorts.

'Change is as good as a holiday,' we say when someone leaves an old job and starts afresh. So often we embrace change. But change comes with a condition in our human standards.

It's OK only if it poses no threat to our security and beliefs.

I think it's fascinating how, when we are young, we can look at other humans as they age and somehow think that it will never happen to us. And when, almost overnight, it starts to happen, we feel shameful or embarrassed. Our society teaches that young is beautiful. And it is. But what about growing old? You almost never see this being advertised or encouraged on TV or in magazines, do you? When you think about it, what a miraculous process it is as we become wiser, care less what others think and need to lean in to other people for support (we'll come back to the value of leaning in, in Chapter 3). Perhaps the lens through which we're viewing it is all wrong.

Just this week I was having lunch with my good mate, Janoah. We have a way of cutting straight to the heart of the matter in things. Our meal hadn't even arrived yet and we had arrived at the conclusion that we (and by that I mean everyone on the planet) are always, at any one point in time, dealing with something. There's always a little hot spot; something that's causing suffering or disturbance of some sort. And it's always when there is some kind of change, or even perhaps lack of change.

Think about it.

What's your current hotspot?

As I write this, mine is loud and clear and becoming more and more obvious visually to others and hormonally to myself. Things are happening in my body. I am, right now, five months' pregnant and from the very beginning of this beautiful journey I started to notice changes. Small things that others wouldn't notice, like bloating from the pregnancy hormones, were a big deal for me. And when I began to thicken around the stomach region this was really scary. I was storing weight in places I never had before and I started to find it hard, a little later down the track, to move around my yoga mat with the same ease I was used to.

What was happening to the body that I had previously been the master of? Was I going to lose myself to being 'the pregnant woman' (which for some reason was really scary for me)?

Sounds crazy, doesn't it? But in my mind, it was very real and totally freaking me out.

But perhaps this needs some background.

As a teenager I was diagnosed with anorexia and after an intervention of sorts I managed to put on enough weight to satisfy the concerns of my parents and friends. I was one of the lucky ones, perhaps. However, anyone who has experienced this illness knows that mentally, it doesn't just go away. And it wasn't until I fell pregnant that I realised just how much of a grip it had on me and how much I still 'controlled' things in my life. Being a healthy-enough weight after high school and all through my early adult life, I was still very disciplined and got away with skipping some of the world's true delights, such as that slice of mud cake and ice cream or a Tim Tam every once in a while, because I was 'healthy'. I was a 'yogi'. I would decline that pasta and take salad and people would say things like, 'Ooh I wish I was that controlled'. Or, 'It's no wonder you look the way you do.' And perhaps this fuelled the lingering anorexic inside. (But if I went into the psychology we'd need another book.)

The point of the story is that falling pregnant has been the biggest blessing, saviour and teacher I've known so far and there isn't a day that goes by that I don't acknowledge the miracle that is conception and pregnancy. It's taught me I can't over-control to the point skipping meals as I used to. I can't skimp on nourishment. I need to look after myself now more than ever before, because it's not just me I'm taking care of anymore. There's a miracle inside me that needs nourishment, love and for me to lead by example.

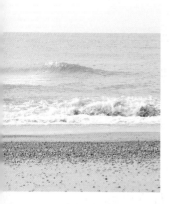

As I write this, five months in, I wouldn't say I'm completely at ease with it yet, but I'm more and more enjoying the process and the changes. I don't mind my belly getting bigger as it's proof that this little girl inside is growing at a healthy rate – it's the other parts that are taking a little more adjustment. The fat that naturally gets stored in places it never used to and the insatiable appetite. But every change is teaching me something. And I'm ridiculously lucky that I have an incredibly supportive partner who loves my new curves.

Perhaps the life lesson regarding impermanence that I'm getting schooled on the most with my pregnancy is this: We can look at change through two lenses. One that teaches us to clamp down, restrict and hold onto what we have for dear life – resisting the flow of life. This one creates only suffering.

Or we can look through the lens that sees us fall back into the flow of life and embrace change. It doesn't mean we can't be scared (fear is natural and sometimes helpful), but that we should be brave enough to go forward, with the natural order. This lens cultivates joy.

There are many Eastern traditions and cultures that celebrate change. They understand this life cycle of beginning, middle and end, and that the end is to be celebrated just as much as the new beginning.

There are Tibetan monks who work on intricately designed sand mandalas for months. They bend over and dedicate their time and love – one grain at a time – until the beauty of the creation is complete. They then cheerfully destroy it in the ultimate celebration of impermanence.

Across the board in Buddhism, all physical and mental events come into being and dissolve. Nothing lasts, everything decays. It's viewed as normal and taught not to be feared. In fact, it's said that Buddha's last words were to the effect that 'All conditioned things are impermanent. Strive on with diligence.' Suffering is not intrinsic to the world of impermanence and truth; rather, suffering occurs only when we cling.

So how do we break the binds of our beliefs that hold us in place and steadily stuck?

How do we just 'go with the flow' and embrace change?

With a lot of practice and a moment-by-moment mindfulness.

And here's the clincher that has helped me. Immensely. Partly because I believe in magic. I have to. It's a part of who I am. And partly because I've experienced it to be true. Here's the idea.

We think we've got it all under control. We have our plans, we set our goals and we set out to achieve them. But what if there's a power, far greater than just you and I – but that conversely is you and I at the same time – that is orchestrating everything? And what if, just maybe, we allowed ourselves to fall into this great mystery or 'flow of life' to see where it might take us?

Are you brave enough to find out?

Little by little, step by step, we lean in. We trust, and we realise that whatever ideas we may have for ourselves, that life force has plans and opportunities far greater than we could ever have imagined for ourselves.

Trust. It's the secret ingredient to a life of love, joy and total liberation.

By practising deep, concentrated mindfulness, we gain insight into the moment-by-moment coming and going of all things. We begin to see that all things, even those things that may seem constant, are forever changing.

own
the
flow

WHAT ARE YOU RESISTING?

Get clear on what it is that's holding you
back and keeping you from riding the flow.
What are your hang ups around change?

Do you have to manipulate situations
so that you don't get hurt?

Does the idea of finding a grey hair feel
like a nightmare?

Are you anxious about moving cities
or job?

What is it that you resist? Or rather – what
situations cause you the most suffering?

Use the following meditation when you're
feeling stuck, over-controlling or going
through big change.

SURRENDERING TO THE FLOW

Find a few minutes to yourself. Five is
great. Ten is ideal. Spend the first few
moments grounding and settling and
then repeat this mantra to yourself:

'I am aware of the universal life force
flowing through me now. I know it. I feel it.
I am it.' After repeating this silently three to
five times, focus on the state of your breath.
Allow it to be relaxed, with no force, and
observe that you are 'being breathed'. It's as
if some mysterious force other than just
you is breathing you.

mantra | love and light

Practise this moving meditation with the intention to move with ease and cultivate a sense of lightness and joy. Think, as you practise this joy on the mat, how you can take it with you into the rest of your day.

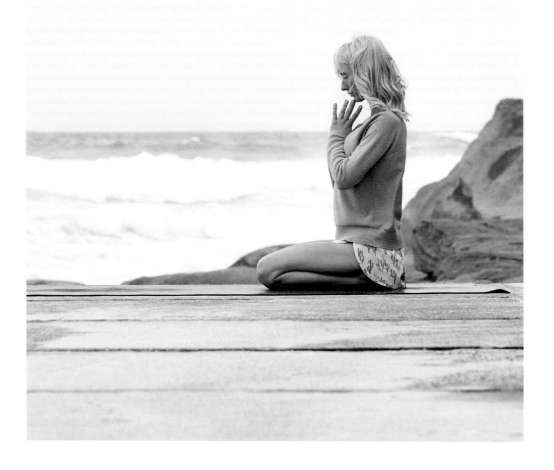

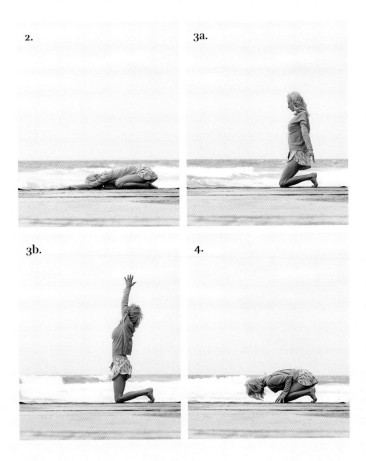

2.

3a.

3b.

4.

Repeat the moving meditation either once each side, or up to eight times, making sure you switch sides each time.

1 Hero's Pose Namaste
Come into a kneeling position with palms together at heart. Close your eyes and feel the rhythm of your breath. Feel the sensation of it move in and out of the nose. Repeat the mantra, 'Love and light', silently to yourself.

2 Child's Pose
From hero's pose, take the hands out in front, stretching your arms out while resting the shoulders down the back. Stay for five to ten breaths to ground and 'arrive' on your mat. Start to breathe in and out of the nose slowly and fluidly. Take this breath awareness with you into this little flow.

3 Sun Flower Salutes
On an inhalation slide the hands in towards you, curl the toes under and come up onto your knees. Raise your arms and look up if it feels comfy on your neck.

4 As you exhale curl into a little ball, cupping the finger tips under the shoulders with the forehead almost on the ground. On the inhalation come up onto the knees again then repeat three times.

5.

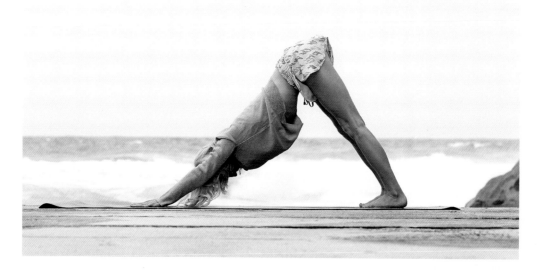

5 Downward Dog
After your fourth sun flower salute, take the hands out in front so you're on all fours, placing the hands just in front of the shoulders. Curl the toes under and lift the knees off the earth as you press the hips up and back. You can soften the knees to lengthen the spine if you feel yourself rounded out or hunched through the shoulders; otherwise press your heels towards the earth. Wrap the outer up edges of arms in towards each other and allow the neck to hang freely from the shoulders. Stay in this first downward dog for five breaths the first time around then just one breath as you move through the next few repeats.

Do the next two postures on the right side first.

6 Three-Legged Dog
From downward dog, firmly and equally press both hands into the earth as you inhale the right leg up and back behind you, keeping both the hips and shoulders square to the ground. Dial your right little toe down to the ground and spread

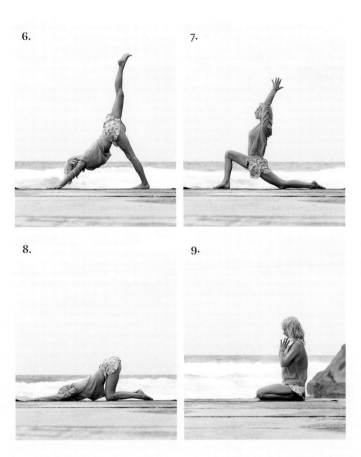

6.

7.

8.

9.

through the toes.
Breath generously.
As you exhale step your
right foot forward into...

7 Psoas Lunge
Step the right foot
through between the
hands, lining up the
right knee and ankle so
the joints are stacked.
To ground and stabilise
for this one, press your

right foot firmly into the
ground as well as the
top of the back foot.
As you inhale take your
arms out to the side and
up above your head with
hands facing each other
and shoulder distance
apart. Inhale to
lengthen the spine and
exhale to ease the hips
down and forward.

**8 Anahatasana
(Melting Heart)**
From the psoas lunge
and on an exhalation,
take the hands down
to frame the right
foot. On an inhalation,
slide (using the strength
of your core) your
right knee back to
meet the left quietly.
Exhale and slide your

hands out in front of
you, keeping hips
over knees.

9 Hero's Pose
Move back to hero's
pose. Stay for five
breaths, then repeat
again with three-legged
dog and psoas lunge
on the left side.

A beautiful lesson in impermanence

This year has been a ride. On the day I heard the news my dad, Michael 'Snowy' Kendall, had died, my partner Andrew and I had just returned home from an overnight Sydney boat stay that he'd bought for me as a Christmas gift. We'd spent the evening being taken around Sydney Harbour on a yacht by a very chatty and friendly captain and then the boat was moored, leaving just the two of us near Mosman. It was a beautiful experience complete with a packed dinner hamper and, at night, being rocked to sleep by the gentle motion of the body of water below.

We woke to a stunning day, popped our cossies on and swam from the boat to the secluded little beach only 20 metres away. For some reason more hesitant of the swim back (a little fearful of what could be under the water), I stayed close behind a much braver Andrew on the return to the boat, where we finished our packed picnic hamper.

We remarked on the beauty around us and felt grateful for the experience. Our hearts opened a little more.

Shortly after, another captain picked us up and took us back to Double Bay, from where we drove our car home.

Being a Monday, when I teach late in the evening and so usually have part of the morning at home to either work in quiet or spend time with Andrew, I took my time getting ready for work then headed in. I was just around the corner from the studio when I got the call from Andrew.

'Something's happened to your dad,' he said, in an unmistakably sombre tone.

I knew immediately what he meant. Dad had been unwell for quite some time and, to be honest, I had sensed his slow fade for a while and knew the life was slowly leaving him. Nonetheless, no one really expected his death to come this soon. Or on this day. But that's part of this beautiful, ever-changing life. It's a mystery. To illustrate the rest of this story and stunning life lesson, I'm sharing with you the eulogy that I read at my father's funeral a few days later.

When we got the news on Monday of Dad dying, I felt at first sad, heart ache-y, dis-believing, grief stricken and cried in waves all day. But towards the evening calm set in and I felt humbled and grounded.

Humbled because it was a reminder of our mortality and how short and precious our lives really are. And grounded because, as I'm sure you all knew with his recent sufferings from a fall and ill health, he was now in a better place. Dad had his weaknesses. We all do. The gravitas of that is heavy but also reminds me of many lessons he taught me. On my 21st birthday when I had a small gathering of close friends at home, he spoke. I can't remember exactly what he said except this, which is crystal clear: 'Follow your heart and pursue what makes you happy.'

When I left my job in advertising to study and teach yoga, a big jump into an unknown future, I heard these words. Whenever I'm challenged with business relationships and standing up for myself, I hear these words. Whenever I knew, in my heart of hearts, that a relationship wasn't right, I heard these words. And they were always backed up with him saying, in his own quiet way, 'You do what's right for you, KJ.' (My middle name is Joanna, and 'KJ' was the nickname Dad used for me from when I was tiny.)

I like to think that any of the success I've had with my career, business relationships and love decisions were inspired by Dad.

They say that when a person dies, all that's left are their purest of qualities. Everything else dissolves. And when I think of Dad's they are:

GENEROUS. WISE. KIND.

We each have our own sweet memories of Dad but here are a few of mine.... an 'ode', if you will, to Dad.

You were the soft touch. Mum was the disciplinary (and by the way, Mum, thank you – because you shaped me into the hard-working, dedicated and confident girl I am today), but Dad, you were the gentle one who listened patiently.

I remember you coming home from the orchards with those funny sock protectors around your ankles, and being down in the sheds skating while you carted apples from one store room to the other.

Banjo playing around the dining room table. Singing Streets of London or telling politically incorrect jokes, all frequently sealed by you falling asleep at the table.

Fawlty Towers. Blackadder. M*A*S*H. Are You Being Served? Tom Clancy novels.

You putting me down your shirt to warm my cold feet as a kid when skiing.

I remember feeling safest at night going to sleep if you were out in your office working away. You being there, my protector, was comforting.

GENEROUS. WISE. KIND.

All these memories I will keep warm and close in my heart, Dad.

Love, your KJ.

———

Those minutes of the eulogy were probably the longest but most heart-felt I've experienced. To truly feel what I felt, to express it in a way that said good bye and to honour his life, as scary as it was to get up and say all of that, makes me so glad I did it.

Death is one of the hardest pills to swallow. When we lose someone we love it's never easy. But again, if we grieve with emotional intelligence – feeling the full spectrum of what we're experiencing and making space for whatever comes up in the process as opposed to numbing through over-use of alcohol, drugs, food or whatever else we can find – we can actually lean into the beauty of it.

We can see through that lens that trusts the flow of life. Death can be a beautiful opportunity to celebrate a life that was, and bring together people who also loved and respected this person. Which brings us to the biggest, brightest and most beautiful thing I've learnt from impermanence – that life is short and to cherish, savour and embrace all your moments.

We all know, in some way, that life is short but quite often it's not until a near-death or fatal event that we truly know it to be true. Abraham Maslow, an often-quoted humanistic psychologist who had a near fatal heart attack, summed it up, saying that his confrontation with death, and his escape from it, made everything feel sacred and precious. He felt the impulse to embrace life and let himself be overwhelmed by it. The ever-present possibility of death, he said, made passionate love more possible.

When you read his thoughts, do you sense that with the possibility of death, love is even more possible? I certainly do.

Part of the ride that this year has been was finding out, shortly before hearing the news of Dad, that I was pregnant. So as one life ended, another began. Isn't that truly magic?

Around the same time this was happening with my father, someone close to me stepped away from me. We had a falling out over a conversation that should have been done and dusted right there and then, or at least a few days after as the dust had settled following my father's wake. But the dip in our relationship involved no conversation

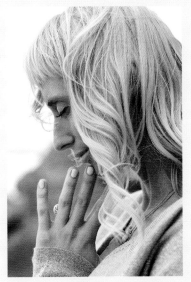

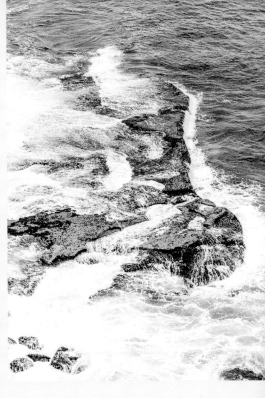

for many weeks and at a time in my life when I really wanted her to be a part of my new pregnancy journey. She wouldn't speak to me. I sent texts, left various voice messages and sent her good vibes through my twice-daily meditations.

What I realised from this is that we all grieve in different ways and that it's important to honour that; to be sensitive in times of grief and to show each other compassion and love. No matter what. Love should lead the way.

Life's too short to go without the people you love for too long. In an instant we can lose someone. I don't want that person to die knowing that I loved them but didn't tell them. I hope this hits *you* in just the right way.

PHILOSOPHY 101.
Stiram Sukham Asanam: equal parts effort to ease

The *Yoga Sutras of Patanjali* are a collection of 196 Indian sutras on the theory and practice of yoga. They were compiled prior to 400 CE. So... they're pretty old and are respected amongst yogic and spiritual scholars alike.

These 'threads' (as sutra translates from the Sanskrit) of wisdom offer guidelines for living a meaningful and purposeful life.

And when you start to explore them, you realise just how far off track we've come with yoga in the modern world. Patanjali, in all of the sutras, rarely mentions the physical postures, what we so commonly think of as 'yoga'. He refers to alignment zero times and mentions no words that come close to flexibility.

Instead the sutras discuss how kleshas (obstacles) can be overcome through meditation, how the practices of yoga can calm the chatter in your mind, how we can live in harmony, and so many other rich philosophical ways of viewing life.

One of the few lines that refers to the physical postures (asanas) goes like this: *Sthira Sukham Asanam*. And that loosely translates to 'The posture should be steady and comfortable'.

So when leading classes I will often talk to the delicate dance between effort and ease. In any posture, take the time to notice if you're over-gripping, over-tensing, over-holding. Or at the other end of the spectrum, are you lethargic, or putting in no effort at all?

And this is relevant to how we live off the mat, and in particular to our relationship to joy.

How can we be alert and attentive and active in this world, while at the same time tender, soft, malleable and open to the opinions, views and approaches of others?

In any one situation, do we over-control, unable to see the value of the opinion of others? Or do we back down and retreat from having an opinion? Do we not 'show up' at all?

Both options kill joy. Really.

Life is a delicate dance between give and take, hold and release.

It's this dance that keeps our awareness of impermanence so alive. If we are able to stay open to each moment, the dance is sweet; it flows, it feels right, and others stand by watching in amazement. It's truly inspiring.

Knowing when to 'let go' and knowing when to 'stand up' and fight for something. Knowing when to hustle (because sometimes we just have to) and knowing when to slow down.

And even better... leading with hustle and heart; now that's a winning combo.

People who have achieved this kind of clarity are usually in tune with themselves. They honour the yin within the yang and the yang within the yin.

They have healthy ideas around boundaries and relationships and they are aligned with their values and vision for wholehearted living.

Stiram Sukham Asanam (also from the sutras), equal parts effort to ease – learning when to hustle or lean into heart – is a practice just like anything else. We don't call it yoga 'practice' for nothing.

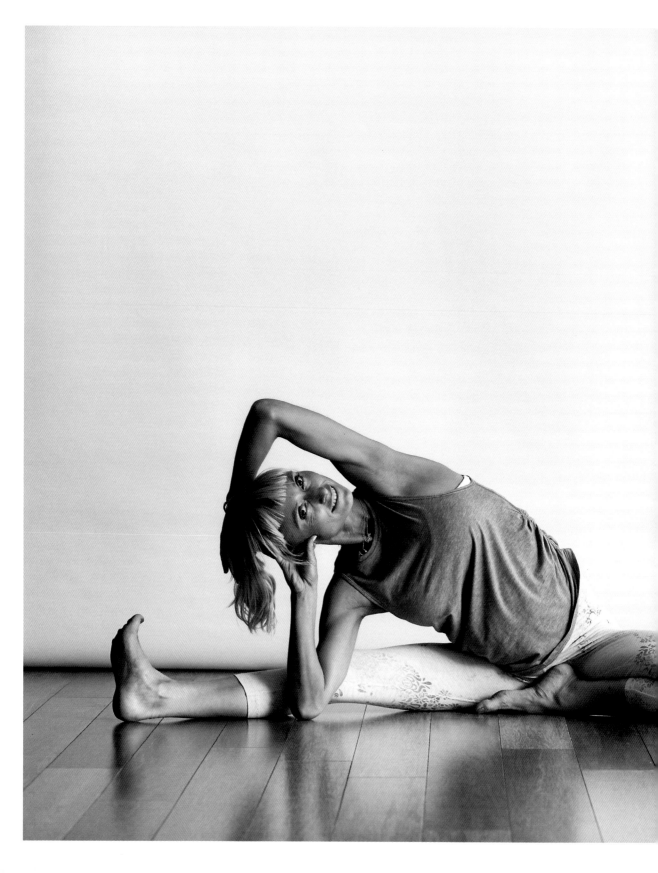

Joy versus happiness

There's a difference.

We all want different things in life, right?

Some of us want fancy cars and others aim to own a shack by the beach. The adventurous types have ambitions to save enough money to travel the world in retirement, while those that like to stay a little closer to home might want to own a business that will sustain a quiet life and a few dogs. Some I know want fame and to mark their place in the world with a loud legacy: be a great mum; be the CEO of the advertising agency they're an employee at; write books; build houses; act; play.

Our aspirations are individual. That's what makes us all unique and gives us all purpose and drive in life.

However it is we aspire to live, there seems to be a common thread.

We want to be 'happy'.

Which is only natural. Who wouldn't?

But what do we really mean when we say we want to be happy? And are we setting the bar high enough?

In the Pali language (a sacred language in some of the religious texts in Hinduism and Buddhism) there are two words for happiness: pamoja and sukha.

Pamoja is the kind of happiness we get in response to someone shooting a perfectly aimed compliment at us. It's the feeling of biting into a sweet, perfectly crunchy apple. It's what we feel when we win a bet or shoot a goal. In other words, it's in response to external stimulus.

Sukha is a little longer-lasting and perhaps deeper. It's feeling happy for no reason. And, as far as I can tell, this is joy.

Psychologists often say that joy and happiness are two different things. Both are wonderful. But joy is the golden child. It is more consistent. It's our true nature, or Buddha nature, and comes from an abundant source within. Joy is revealed when you're at peace with yourself.

Happiness tends to be externally triggered and is felt in reaction to other people, places and events. If everything goes according to your expectations and standards, you're happy. But if things don't go to plan, that happiness is jeopardised.

Joy, however, is being happy for no reason. It's an understanding that no matter what – whether things work out or not – you can still choose to be happy.

And when we choose to live in joy, we can expect the following to happen:

We sweat the small stuff less.

We're optimistic.

We go with the flow and trust the mystical ride of life – the ups and downs... all of it.

We're inspiring to others.

So I don't want to just be happy in life. I want to be joy-FULL.

How about you?

Joy – you can't fake it.

Lean in a little. Listen up.

A universal truth.

We can't just 'pretend' a state of joy when what we really need to do is feel the sad.

I used to think that you could fake your way to joy. That if you just pretended to be in a good head space, repeated diligently your positive affirmations and did good by others, you'd eventually get there.

And I think that's partly true.

We can definitely create an 'atmosphere' for joy by making sure we set aside time for those things that we know bring us joy and in doing so, attract more joy. And actually pamoja – the external causes of happiness – can create an environment for sukha – joy and delight – to show up more frequently.

But ultimately there will always be emotions that are blocking the way and when these show up, quite often the only way through to the joy is to feel our way through those other, 'not so nice' emotions.

The first step is to stop labelling the 'not-so-nice' feelings as good or bad, naughty or nice. They're just feelings.

This takes practice, discipline and an unwavering remembrance that it's all worth it; that it's building resilience and willpower.

According to Buddhist beliefs, our natural state is 'Buddha Nature', which is one of pure joy and pure consciousness.

So let's imagine your joy as the sky.

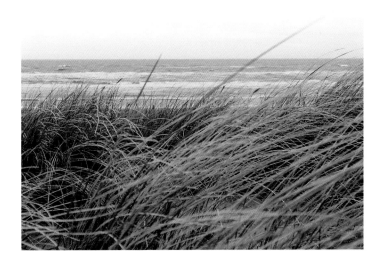

As you look at it, some days the sky is clear and blue and vast. Others it's cloudy and grey, sometimes stormy with lightning, hail or snow. But ultimately, we know that behind the weather, there's the sky. Always. It hasn't gone anyway, sometimes it's just covered up.

The weather generally passes and we remember how it feels to be clear, blue and vast again.

And how much do we appreciate the blue sky after a week of rain?

Like the weather, we can't really stop our emotions. They're going to come and go. We can, however, go with them, feel what we need to feel through them and release them when they've run their course.

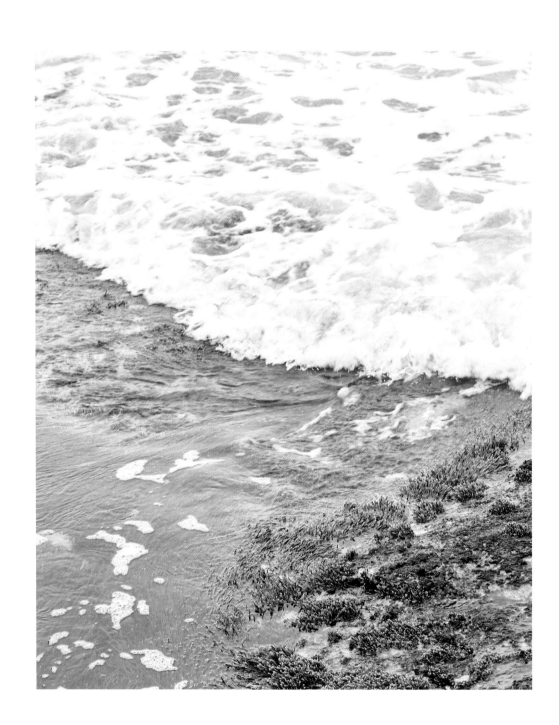

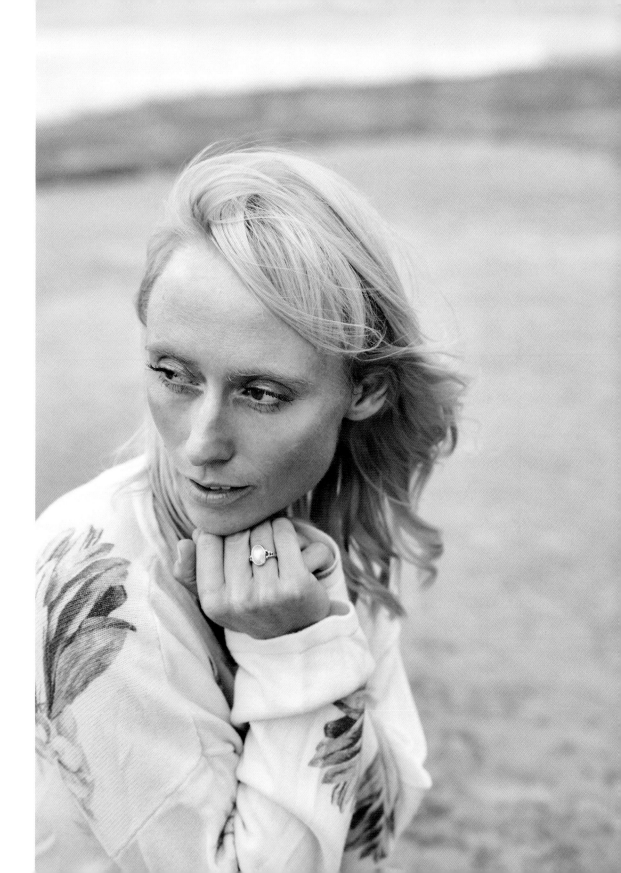

Feel what you feel

It's a universal truth that when we choose (and there's always a choice) to numb grief, sadness or pain of any kind we automatically, in doing so, numb the joy, love and elation.

Being whole is being open to all the emotions that arise.

So how do we numb?

We over-eat, over-drink, over-do. We get busy, procrastinate, play ourselves down, take prescription drugs, recreational drugs. We blame, rage, retreat and generally hide from our feelings in all kinds of ways. These are just a few.

And this is why slowing down is such a relevant step in recognising what it is we're numbing and how we numb.

I remember being on one of those speeding bullet trains in Japan on an early adulthood adventure. Sure, it was new and thrilling and quite a fun experience and it was relatively easy to make out what we were passing in the distance, houses, other buildings and trees, but the things that were up close were a blur. The form barely existed before it flew past.

This is what we do with our emotions. The ones that are most challenging to lean into, we tend to speed through, skim over and barely acknowledge. We use our coping skills of choice to numb what's really going on up close.

And then, because we're used to running at such a pace and the momentum has built (and perhaps because the numbing becomes comfortable after some time), we miss all the delicious emotions that come our way and that get close.

So.

If we truly want to feel deeply, and I think we all do – we all want to experience the full range of human emotions because that's what it means to be whole, that's what it means to live wholeheartedly – we have to start paying attention to, and acknowledging, each sensation or emotion as it arises.

This concept of 'feeling what you feel' comes into my teaching in almost every class. I encourage students to start an inner dialogue that uses not words but rather sensation. Thoughts and words can mislead – the body rarely lies.

Your cells are full of wisdom if only you'd lean in and listen.

And it's this deep listening, attentive to not only the sensations that arise but also the feelings and emotions, that keeps us in flow and in synch with the natural rhythms of the body and their ability to move feelings and emotions.

We have one of two decisions to make when, on the mat, we come up against resistance and what one of my teachers, Sarah Powers, calls 'interesting' sensations. By this she means the ones that are uncomfortable. We don't want them to be risky to the point that we injure ourselves through over-effort, but rather a place where we greet an 'edge'.

We can choose to numb. We can avert our attention to what's going on around us in the room by looking at the tights on the girl next to us or checking on our pedicure or tip toe-ing out of the room mentally onto plans for breakfast or work.

Or we can choose to stay. In staying, we're brave enough to go right to that epicentre of sensation, and not only ride the breath consciously in and out but use it to release and move tension.

The inhalation can often highlight the sensation and bring it right to the surface, whilst the exhalation provides the opportunity for you to release and soften.

You always have a choice. Go. Or stay.

Emotions are just like sensations. They move. But only if you're willing to stay.

And because what we practise on the mat, we take with us off the mat, the asana practice can develop your skills in intelligently processing things as they arise, not sweating the small stuff, and remaining calm and patient no matter what comes up.

This was one of the very first things I noticed when I took up the practice. Quite quickly, we're talking within weeks, I noticed that I was less agitated with myself and others and way more relaxed. My focus improved and my sleep went next level. The quality of it was better because I was 'releasing' often.

Yogi 2

There's a pretty special soul in my life. Her name's Maryanne and she's part of our epic teaching team at Flow Athletic. She's a blessing and the yin to my yang.

Maryanne is one of the most level, open, accepting, non-judgemental and kind-hearted people I know. I call her 'Peace Angel'.

Does it mean she doesn't get angry? No. She rarely does but when she does you know it's for a worthy cause. She's not easily ruffled nor offended.

She's joyful and has a wicked sense of humour.

And when she's in the middle of a break up, she makes space to truly feel what she's feeling. And you know what? As much as it hurts her like the rest of us, she knows that the sorrow is 'the way through'. And she marvels in the beauty of the process. She knows, on some deep level, that at the other end of sorrow is something special; more sparkling; more vibrant.

She makes me want to be a better human: softer, lighter, all-in.

The 90-second rule

American neuroscientist and speaker Jill Bolte Taylor wrote a book titled *A Brain Scientist's Personal Journey*. In it, she explains that the physiological basis of anger only lasts 90 seconds. When we get angry, she says, the chemicals released by the brain surge through our body. But that's it – if we're angry after those 90 seconds, it's because we've chosen to let that circuit continue to run.

All emotions last for less than 90 seconds, Taylor explains. If anything continues after that it is because we have added our own story and chosen to hold on to the emotion. When we replay the memory that is attached to a thought, or repeat one of our old painful stories, we remain caught in the cycle and it will get more and more difficult to disconnect.

According to Taylor, if we are aware that emotions take 90 seconds to surge through our systems we can simply allow them to naturally pass and flush out. If we choose to fight the emotion we will emphasise it further and then we will need to fight it again and again, and by then the emotion will have the power to control us.

There's a tool that we can use within this 90-second period, one I've learnt in mindfulness, which uses the acronym RAIN.

We **recognise** that we're having an emotion and gently turn towards what we're experiencing. It may be helpful to name the emotion. E.g. I am overwhelmed, outraged, heartbroken.

We then **allow** it to be. It's as if we 'make space' for it to exist. This alone can soften the emotion or feelings that are coming up. Allowing doesn't mean you are giving up, it just means you're dissolving the resistance that can cause the emotion to get stuck. Allowing is also saying 'yes' to the moment.

Quite often the recognising and allowing are enough but sometimes the emotion will lend itself to a desire to **investigate**. You can investigate by asking questions such as 'Why do I feel like this?'; 'Did I get enough sleep last night?'; 'Is this actually worth getting anxious over?'; and 'Could I relax and let this go?'. It's important not to spend too much time on this step.

The final step is to **nurture**. And this one makes such a difference to how we experience and, hopefully, let go of the emotion or situation at hand. It's relevant to note that sometimes emotions are there to protect us and are biological. It's not your fault that you react with fear. So to nurture would be to address or communicate with the emotion directly, thank it even, and say that for today, you won't need it. Sometimes emotions, just like our children and friends, want to be recognised. And this can soften everything.

And what happens after the rain?

Often there's an abundance of lush life; a sweet flow of energy and a new sense of expansiveness.

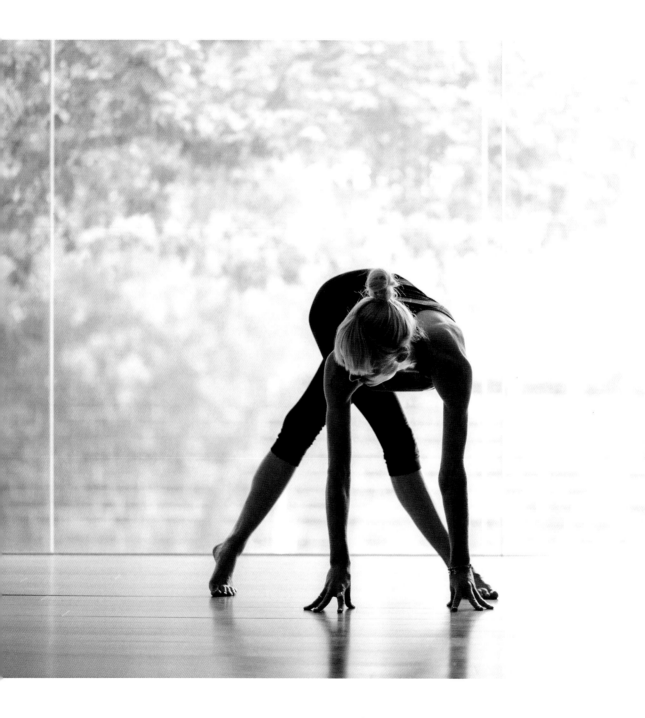

own
the
flow

LET IT RAIN

Next time you have an emotion come up
and you feel like reacting in some way, take
a comfortable seat or stand still and go
through your grounding ritual. Feel the Earth
underfoot, breathe conscious breaths and
locate where the emotion is sitting in your
body. Allow your awareness to rest right
there and for 90 seconds continue to breath
and go through the four-point RAIN process.

Recognise the emotion or feeling and
where it's manifesting in the body.

Allow or even 'accept' and make space
for what you're feeling.

Investigate and enquire into why you're
feeling what you're feeling.

Nurture and be kind to yourself. Try not
to beat yourself up for feeling this way
and know that all emotions are relevant.

My mentor, Michael Trembath, would also
say to soften that place where you feel the
tension and watch it move in a downwards
flow out of the body.

Gratitude

Why practise gratitude? Because simply put...

Whatever we appreciate, appreciates.

What we give thanks for only generates more of the energy of that thing that we're appreciating.

Plus. Each time we 'give thanks' and acknowledge something, magic happens. We rise, energetically, to a higher vibration. All through the power of gratitude.

Research has shown that expressing daily gratitude can increase your happiness by up to 25 per cent. That's definitely enough of a reason for me.[1,2] So even if you're feeling down in the dumps or can't seem to shift a mood no matter how much sitting with it you do, find something to be grateful for. It can be anything from coffee to your cat.

I practise gratitude at the end of each of my yoga classes. I place my awareness in the heart and allow anything I feel grateful for to come into my mind. Rather than searching for things to be grateful for (this can make the practice of gratitude feel like a chore), let things come to you. Sometimes you might need to clear more space and stillness to let them arise. Perhaps one day it's one thing and then next 10.

Do it.

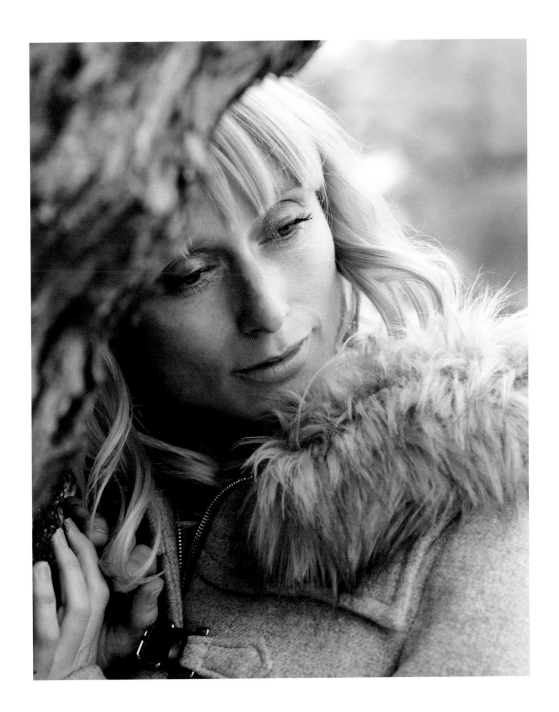

"When you arise in the morning, think of what a precious privilege it is to be alive – to breathe, to think, to enjoy, to love."

Marcus Aurelius,
Roman Emperor, 121–180 AD

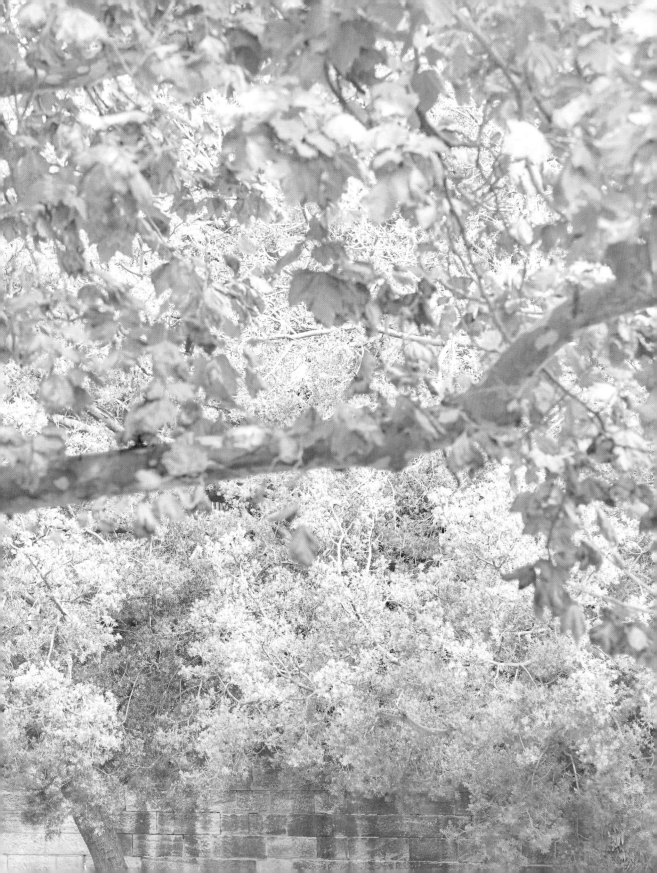

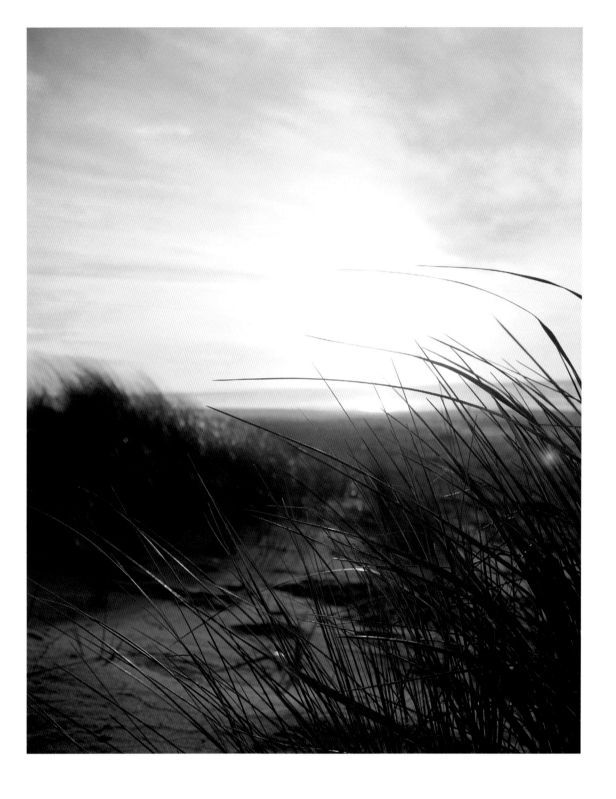

own
the
flow

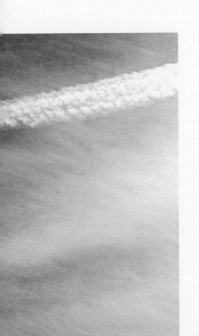

GIVE GRATITUDE

Today, start a gratitude list. Go ahead.
What are you grateful for today?

At first this may seem forced and like
you're hustling to find things to be grateful
for, but after you spend some time just
writing what comes up for you, you'll find
the flow. So, don't go searching, let the
gratitude come to you.

Some days the big stuff comes up – like the
deep connection I have with my partner,
my health, my mum, the gorgeous group of
supportive and loving friends around me,
the roof over my head and the comfy bed
we sleep in each night, beautiful Bronte
Beach, my business partner, Benny, and all
of his guidance and loyalty. Other days it's
threaded with the seemingly smaller stuff
like my morning coffee, the sweet barista
who smiles as she hands it over, the
delicious breakfast slice I have every
Saturday morning on the way to teach
classes, my car, the fact that I have money
enough to pay the bills as they come in.

It doesn't matter how big or small, it all
counts to the quality of your vibration.

Follow the charm

I first heard the expression 'Follow the charm' when I did a course in Vedic meditation. During the week-long course I was 'inducted', in a sense, into the tradition through a ceremony held by my teacher and the receiving of an individualised mantra, followed by explanations and talks on the Vedic meditation tradition, as well as being led through a meditation, so that by the end of the course I could practise anywhere, anytime, twice a day for 20 minutes.

It's been a game changer. The Vedic tradition is full of beautiful philosophies, sayings and notions but the one that stands out the most to me is 'Follow the charm'.

The charm is what pulls you. It's like a diamond sparkling from afar or the sun sparkling on the ocean. We can't help but look and be lured. Same goes for desires.

Ever felt so deeply connected, rested or clear minded that you get a brilliant idea in a flash? Or the urge to do something really tugs at your heart? This is the charm.

And in the Vedic tradition, the notion is to gravitate towards that which pulls you. Because it cultivates more joy.

Think of the charm as leaving little breadcrumbs and hints along your quest for the life you're destined to have.

An opportunity may come out of nowhere and you feel 'charmed' by it. It's clearly an indication to follow, stay curious and watch.

The charm doesn't always lead us towards what we'd call a desirable outcome, but there's always a teaching in it, a silver lining. Let's not confuse following the charm with being lazy or over-indulging in things that, in the long run, are no good for us. For example, we could say that we feel way more pulled to lying on the sofa all day instead of taking 20 minutes to go to a yoga class or lift some weights at the gym. Or we could say we're lured towards smoking cigarettes, which in the long run can lead to illness and even death.

And let's not confuse betrayal with charm either – for example, you have a strong physical urge to get back together with your ex when you know in your heart of hearts that doing so is a betrayal of self.

Charm is way more magical.

It lights you up, tugs on your heart strings and pulls you in. It may seem mysterious. It could be something where to follow it would be to take a leap of faith or a leap in logic.

It's about doing what feels right, true and good. It gives clarity around what you're meant to be doing in this world as a conscious, awake and wholehearted person. It's like following nature's cues as to 'where next'? You don't have to know how to get to where you're going. You just follow the charm. One step at a time. When we look back on our lives to reflect on the steps that got us to where we are, we'll see a series of charms; little doors that we had a choice to walk through.

When I look at it like that, it feels like magic. We think we have a grand plan on how to get somewhere but, really, each day we're being presented with a series of choices. Ultimately, we don't know what's on the other side. We just trust the gut feeling.

Follow the charm.

And, as if we need another incentive to live in our most joyous state, this is the place where these charming moments occur most frequently. Joy is magic. And 'only always' makes space for more joy. There's no cap on our joy, just as there is no cap on the amount of charming moments you get in one lifetime.

CHAPTER 3

Connection

leaning in.
to you, to others.

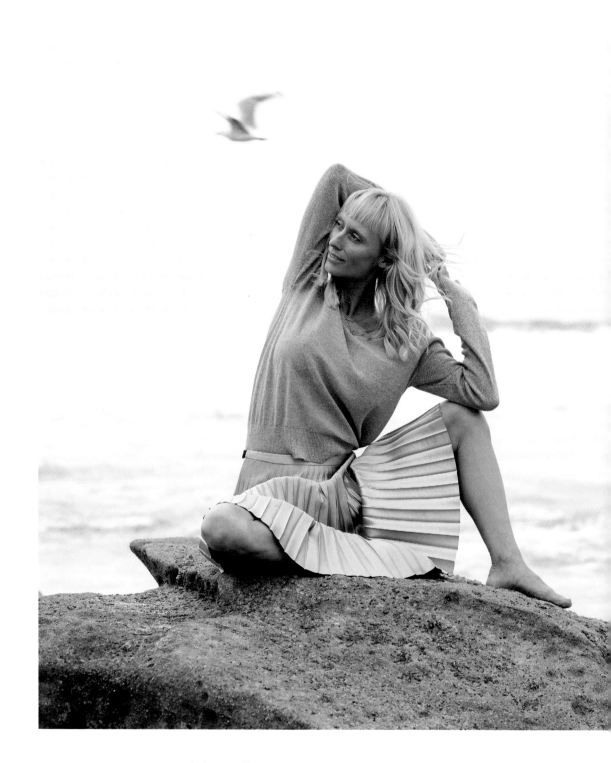

MANTRA:

COOL,
CALM,
CONNECTED

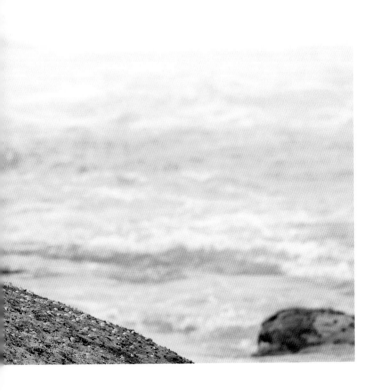

"We cannot live only for ourselves. A thousand fibres connect us with our fellow men."

Herman Melville, American author and playwright, 1819–1891

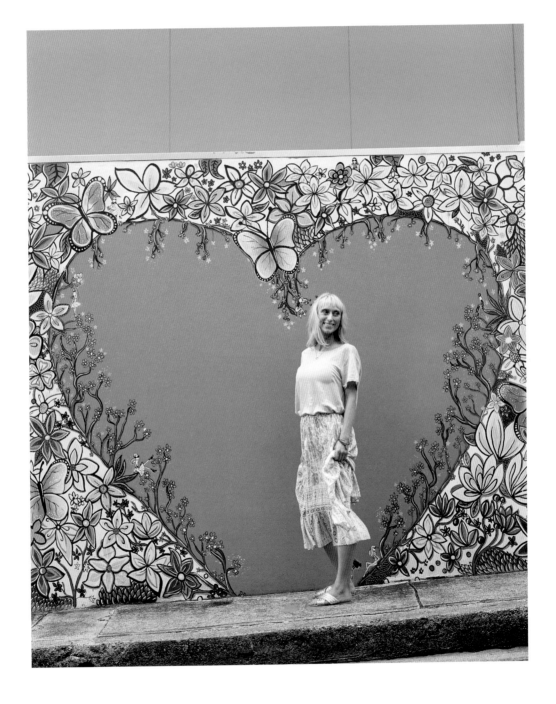

Connection.

It's why we're here.

It's what warms the heart.

It's the foundation of family, loyalty and togetherness.

It challenges you and makes you a better human.

It's what scares you, lights you up and totally pulls you down.

Real connection. Deep-down, authentic spirit-to-spirit connection is what teaches us that there is no separation between you and me. That we're all made up of the same stuff. We all hurt, we all love and we all go through things.

Connection has the capacity to blow your heart wide open and fear of connection can close your heart right down.

To allow yourself to really connect, to truly be seen and to truly see others...

Now that's the kind of connection I want to experience. Often.

In an era where we have more than enough ways (perhaps too many) to connect, why is it that we feel so disconnected? Why don't we experience that deep-down, heart-felt connection with more of the people around us?

I truly believe that it's possible. I don't believe we were designed to personally (in a one-on-one kind of way) connect with every human on the planet and there's both science and ancestral reasons for that, which I'd love you to read about later in this chapter, but I do believe that we can have connection with those around us and in particular, those closest to us more often.

When we choose to live in flow, we arouse a vibration within ourselves that makes us more open, alert, alive and appreciative of the world around us – including the people. When we're insular, closed off and disconnected from others, there's little chance of a heart spark or the genuine connection you get when looking into a stranger's eyes.

When we're in flow, we attract positive situations and people.

It's a universal law. And when we, collectively, are in flow we thrive as communities.

I remember being on holiday with my partner. This particular day he'd skipped a surf to come to yoga with me. Upon leaving the little yoga shala in the beautiful village of Princeville on the island of Kauai, he said, 'The world would be a better place if there were more yogis.' To which I simply said, 'yes'. And was secretly chuffed that my boisterous babe was leaning into the way of the yogi. One of my greatest joys.

And I totally agree with him. Naturally. If more people took the time to focus on making connections, the world would be more peaceful. But yoga is just a vehicle. Some of us find a deep-down connection with our inner selves through mountain biking, skiing, surfing, walking, running, knitting, riding horses or baking cakes.

If it lights you up and, when you're doing it, makes you feel like time stands still, that's connection. And when we're more connected to ourselves, we're way more connected, empathetic and compassionate with others.

Every so often, I host yoga retreats. When students arrive the energy is very different to how things are at the end of their visit. Upon arrival, and especially in a group where people are unfamiliar with each other, I'll notice guarded body language and lack of eye

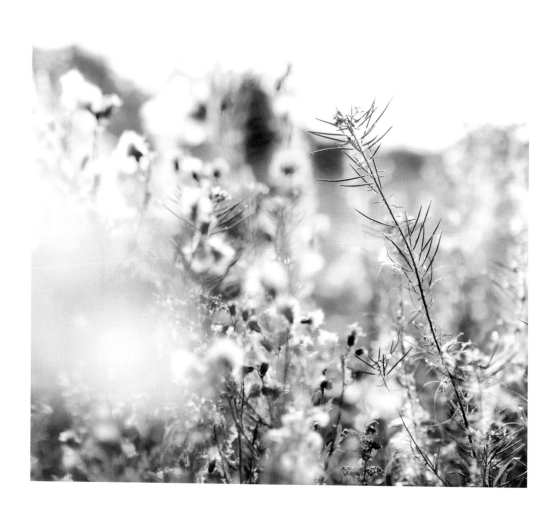

contact. Often, there's a general tendency to quietness or over-the-top interactions. In other words, we generally shrink back or over-perform – both normal human survival techniques.

After a long weekend or a whole week (even better!) the group, when saying farewell or taking part in a closing circle, warmly embrace and look each other in the eyes. They really listen to what others have to say and are conscious of their own words.

And the secret? It's simple. A few days away from work, limited or no time on technology of any kind, good food and plenty of communing with nature. If we really want to get deep, deep down to bring a group together, we might pepper into their routine a group activity in which they are encouraged to get a little (or a lot) vulnerable. It's always up to the practitioner and a facilitator should never push.

But here's what happens. As soon as one person shows their vulnerability – that they're human and that they hurt just like all the others in the group; that they have insecurities about how they're perceived, how much money they have in the bank, whether or not they're good-looking enough, tall enough, skinny enough – it softens the energy in the group and encourages others to crack open.

It's so touching to watch, and to be a part of. When we truly let ourselves be seen is when the deepest of connections take place.

So let's really lean in. Let's discover the parts of ourselves that we don't dare to share. And share them. At first, it's scary. But then you feel lit up and liberated. Let's lean into our connection with others and remember we all have the ability to break down barriers and lift the veils that have kept us from connecting.

Here's to more authentic conversations, heart-felt connections and big love.

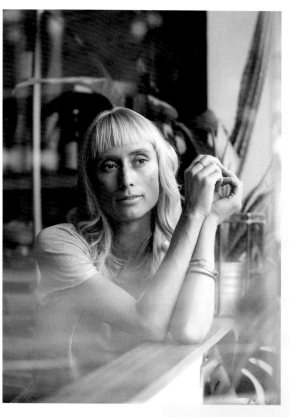

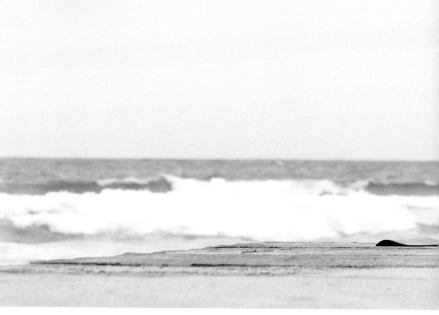

Tribe

And why we struggle to live in large cities

I can be walking through the bustling centre of Sydney and feel as though I'm the only person there.

Head down, gaze down, game face on.

This was me five years ago.

And the internal dialogue went something like this: 'Don't look them in the eye. They might want to stop and say hi and I don't have time for small talk.'

Where are we all going? Why are we in such a rush and when did it become weird to look someone in the eye or say hello?

It's a shame. Now that I've learnt to slow down (well, for the most part) and create more meaningful connections, I realise how cold life is when we are disconnected.

And even now that I have the tools to slow down, it often takes me a few weeks of stress and 'un-doing' to realise that I'm back on the road to burn out.

As I write, right now, I've taken myself down the South Coast of New South Wales not only to craft these words, but also to teach a few classes for a dear friend, Chelsea, who is running a retreat down here.

The night leading up to my trip I got home to the apartment I share with my partner and his nine-year-old – both of whom I love to bits –

and with Andrew at work and Louis camping with a friend's family for school holidays, I was hit with this powerful sense of loneliness. 'Since when did I get so bad at being by myself?' I thought. 'I used to be good at this'.

Upon reflection, I realised that it wasn't that I really felt like I was alone or that I couldn't talk to anyone. I could have picked up the phone to call any one of my close friends and all would have been good. The issue, I realised, was that I had spent the past few weeks in a state of stress and 'doing', so when I had this time by myself, it was a little bit disturbing. I wondered what to do with myself. With the prospect of time alone, and stopping to do nothing, some old mental chatter began to surface: 'Am I being lazy? Am I enough? Should I be doing something productive right now?' The inner chatter showed up as anxiety and a big messy ball of tightness, right below my sternum – an old favourite hideout for it.

And as soon as Andrew walked in the door, the tension melted away and my heart widened. I was once again present and 'at home' in my body. What was this saying about my capacity to be alone when things feel overwhelming?

In this moment, I leave the body. It doesn't feel like a safe place to be when truths come up, so I 'leave'. And although nothing particularly dark was happening at the time, I don't think I'd slowed down for long enough to process everything I had been doing. It was like an overload on my nervous system, which didn't how to deal with it – so its reaction was to freak out and run fear through my body.

As I started driving out of the city the next day and down the beautiful coastline, taking in stunning views of our incredible ocean and beaches, the residual tension from the past few weeks began to dissolve and within twelve hours I was 'back' again, back at home in my body.

I often think about our earliest civilisations and how, yes, life would have been hard (being chased by sabre-toothed tigers and all – no thanks!) but life would have been less complex. Surely.

I know it's not realistic for most of us to jet off on retreat or hit the coast at the drop of the hat. These little spells are truly restorative, but what's more required is our ability to feel at ease and 'at home' in our bodies even in our urban landscapes.

When we look back at the history of the human race, we know that we weren't the only species that existed back in what I call our 'Cave Man' days. Some of those species did not survive. So how did we survive?

Because we worked together.

The only way we could get enough food and protect ourselves was to work together.

When we look at the structure of those early communities, or at least at the 'best guess' by archaeologists and other researchers, everyone had a role[1].

These societies were largely dependent on foraging and hunting. These small bands of hunter-gatherers lived, worked and migrated together before the advent of agriculture. They created their own culture of learned human behaviours that were often linked to survival. Individually, yes, but also as a group.

Trust was cultivated when everyone played their part, contributed (and in return gained fulfilment) and supported the person next to them.

The strongest and fittest of us thrived and got creative in the way we lived: we evolved. Eventually with the expansion of the human population, the size and density of groups increased too.

This often brought with it conflict and competition over the best land and resources. Due to the constraints of available natural resources, these early communities were not very large, but they included enough members to facilitate some degree of the division of labour.

When I think of these early humans, I imagine everyone going about their daily routine, productive in their role and at the end of the day, feeling a sense of community – a satisfaction that each person had fulfilled their role – and ultimately, fulfilled in themselves. I could be just assuming these feelings based on my own experience... but stay with me.

At the end of each day, after meals had been made – a collaboration around the camp fire – and consumed, they would retire to the same cave or site together, to sleep side by side. This was safer – providing more of a chance of survival if a sabre-toothed tiger were to join the group in the middle of the night!

They woke up together. Ate together. Hunted. Gathered. Fought. Rested. Played. Grew up. Made love. Gave birth. Died. Grieved. Celebrated. Even if you didn't particularly like the person next to you from time to time or they rubbed you up the wrong way because they took your last handful of seed when you were starving, you were connected by deep loyalty. An unbreakable bond that meant if you were being dragged down a rapid creek likely to drown, the person next to you would jump in to save you.

All of life's experiences were shared and supported by these small communities. There has to have been a real 'togetherness'. And I still get a sense of this in the small country towns that I visit – including the one I grew up in.

Look at how we've evolved. How clever and great at survival are we!

We now drive around in man-made automobiles, travel to destinations far away and have more than enough means of communication. We've built huge cities designed to house millions of people. We really must applaud ourselves. However, we're still, at the most basic of levels, not that dissimilar to 'back then'. And living in these big cities takes its toll.

Where once we thrived in smaller communities, everyone playing their important role, we now live in a society where to feel we're contributing, we often think we have to achieve and hustle, sometimes to the point of burn-out. I'm talking especially to the A-type over-achiever inside many of us.

It's no wonder we feel unimportant and disconnected, especially when we're so frequently comparing ourselves with others and the seemingly perfect lives they share on social media. We've forgotten something critical and simple. We are enough. You. Me. Just as we are.

Everything about the human body is designed for survival. And still is. Our eyebrows are exactly where they are to keep sweat out of eyes when hunting, sometimes for hours. Our tongues are fine-tuned to taste when something is 'spoiled' and may harm us. Even the way we 'feel' is designed to help us survive. When we feel a connection, a deep-down bond with someone, we know that we can trust them and sometimes even co-create with them. But that comes from time together, loyalty, trust and a depth contributed to by both.

And although it's true we no longer need to hunt for food (instead it's delivered to our door in minutes) and we trust that produce, when bought from the supermarket shelf or the farmer's market, is neither off nor poisonous, we have forgotten something important. We ignore sensations, swallow our feelings and numb ourselves as never before. Half the time our heads are buried in our phones or caught up 'doing', and we deny those ancestral bonds. It's a shame, because they are designed for the health of the 'all', not to mention our capacity to feel real love.

But it's not all doomsday.

I think we can have our cake and eat it too. I think we can use all that modern man has produced, including iPhones, fancy cars (bravo to the eco ones), skyscrapers and drones, but be conscious of our relationship with them. We can continue to live in these big cities that we adore (NYC is my favourite) and make strong and supportive sub-cultures in our local areas.

All of this does happen. There is, around us, living proof that we can build greater bonds and deeper connections.

As more conscious beings do their work in the world (that's you and I!) there's a shift towards remembering.

Remembering what's truly important. Remembering that dates with mates are best prioritised over dates with deadlines. Remembering the medicine of a good belly laugh or a deep, conscious breath. Remembering that the person next to you is just like you and needs all the things that you need to survive: connections, recognition and human touch. It's not all just warm and fuzzies. It's part of our survival. It's genetic. It's called being human.

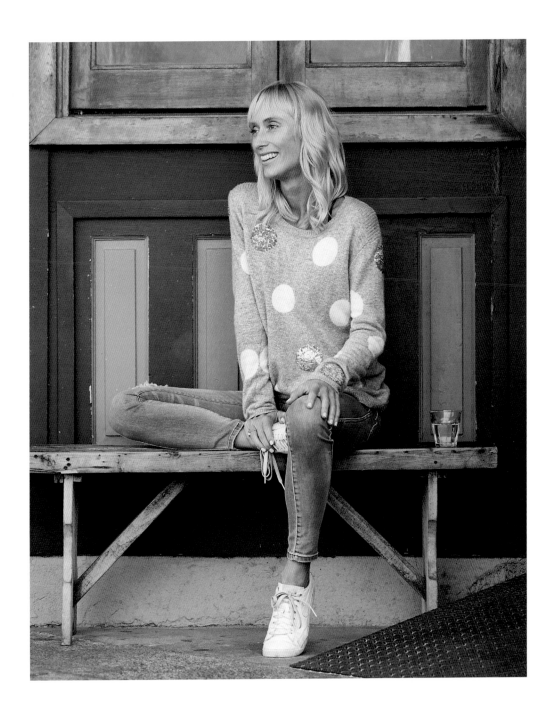

The chemistry of connecting

When it comes to the human body, there's not one part of it that doesn't fascinate me.

Did you know...

Nerve impulses sent from the brain move at speeds of more than 300 kilometres per hour.[2]

The human heart beats up to 100,000 times a day.[3]

A kiss can reduce your stress levels.[4]

The human eye can distinguish more than two million different colours – possibly as many as 40 million.[5]

Everything about us is designed to keep us alive and safe. And for the most part, these goings-on are automated. We go about our day not even having to think about it.

Even the way we 'feel' has a purpose.

If you've ever had feelings of status, pride, confidence, joy or love through connecting with others, chances are it's your body's way of rewarding you. And quite often the feeling 'states' we get into as a result are felt so that we collaborate and work together..

Our bodies want us to connect to each other. Helping others is natural and when the environment is right, that's exactly what happens.

To illustrate our connection chemistry and how it keeps us alive and functioning, as well as keeping us together as small groups or communities (from way back in the day), let's take a playful look at the chemicals in your body.

We have four main feel-good chemicals.[6]

The first two are the endorphins and dopamine. I remember hearing author of *Start with Why*, Simon Sinek, refer to these two as selfish chemicals, because we don't need anyone else to produce them.

*Endorphins have one main job —
to mask physical pain.*

You go for a tough gym session and push hard. Afterwards you feel awesome, right? You've worked your body to a pulp and should hurt, but our bodies hide the pain associated with the 'pushing' so we keep working. Seems crazy, right? Why does this happen? If we look back to our ancestry, we needed to have endurance to hunt food.

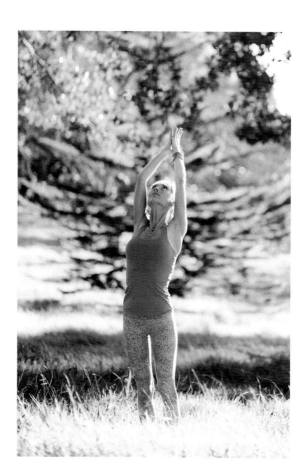
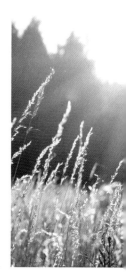

We could literally track a wild animal for hours upon hours until we got a 'kill' to take home to the tribe.

In our modern world, one of the most common times that endorphins get released is during a workout. And that's still a good enough incentive to keep training or practising.

Dopamine is produced to encourage us to keep going. You know that feeling when you cross something off your to do list? That's your body releasing dopamine. Or that feeling when you reach a milestone or goal? That's dopamine.

It's why we're always told to write down our goals, because it feels like we've accomplished something when we cross things off. It's fulfilling and we, as humans, have historically used that feeling to survive. When our early ancestors were foraging for food, for example, dopamine would have helped them focus on that goal. As they got closer to that fruit-filled tree they'd have received a shot of dopamine. Closer again, another shot and another, until 'bam'. They reached the tree and got a huge shot of dopamine.

This is also why leaders share with us a vision.

If we can't see something it's hard to go after it, right? We need to imagine it and set a path to achieve it. Every time we achieve one of those milestones that get us closer to the vision, dopamine is released.

And perhaps because we don't have to forage so much anymore, we replace it with other things. Because the thing about dopamine is this… it's highly addictive.

Shopping, smoking cigarettes and gambling all release dopamine. All can be addictive, right?

Think of your phone. The buzz, the flash, the ring tone, the message tone, the email alert – it's addictive, even if the 'ding' just creates more work for you. When we hear those sounds, we get a hit of dopamine.

'Someone loves us.'

Every time you get a like on Facebook or Instagram – that releases a shot of dopamine.

See how it works?

It's lucky, in this day and age, that we have the other two chemicals, serotonin and oxytocin – the social chemicals.

Serotonin plays many roles, but I think of it as what we get when we feel a sense of pride or accomplishment.

Have you ever achieved something for your community? Were you made the school or sports captain? Perhaps you graduated from university and made a special day of it.

When you get up to receive that accolade and listen to the clapping and cheering around you, your body releases serotonin. It raises not only your sense of pride but confidence. That chemical is rewarding you for your excellence – for leading others, for doing something good for you and your community (your tribe).

The cool thing about this one is that just as you're getting that award or any kind of recognition, those who love and support you are also getting a shot of serotonin.

This chemical is encouraging us to build community. The value of group living is important. We need leaders. We have always lived in hierarchical communities and there will always be people whose status is higher than others.

However, if you are a leader and enjoying all the perks of this kind of status, the group expects you to stand up and lead. You must be willing to rush towards danger to protect your people – be you the captain of the hockey team, the leader of the free world or the leader of your small tribe. A leader must be prepared to sacrifice.

And then there's my favourite feel-good chemical.

Oxytocin is responsible for feelings of love and trust, and encourages us to look after each other.

You get it from bonding. From hugging, kissing, sex – all those feelings of warmth or closeness. And it's what's released, in abundance, in both mother and father when a baby is born.

Quite obviously it's oxytocin that is key for our survival and to maintaining the population.

Acts of generosity and kindness also produce oxytocin. You're walking along a busy city street and the person in front of you drops their wallet without noticing. They're about to walk off so you pick it up and call out to them. Pretty small act of kindness and most people would have done the same in that situation, right? But that person still thinks it's cool and gets a shot of oxytocin. As do you. As does anyone looking on. That brief point of contact between strangers can have a profound effect on anyone looking on.

You spend your Sunday giving up your time at a soup kitchen for homeless people – that generates oxytocin. You go to someone's house for dinner and the very next day you send them a note to say thank you. Oxytocin again.

When we do things for each other, we're rewarded with good vibes. It's all about time, generosity and kindness.

The way we feel is 'only always' telling us something. It pays to lean in and listen.

Knowing the difference between a habit or addiction and the more sustainable and healthy feel-good hormones is a skill.

Although we don't need to hunt and forage for food in the way we used to, that basic need for human connection is still relevant.

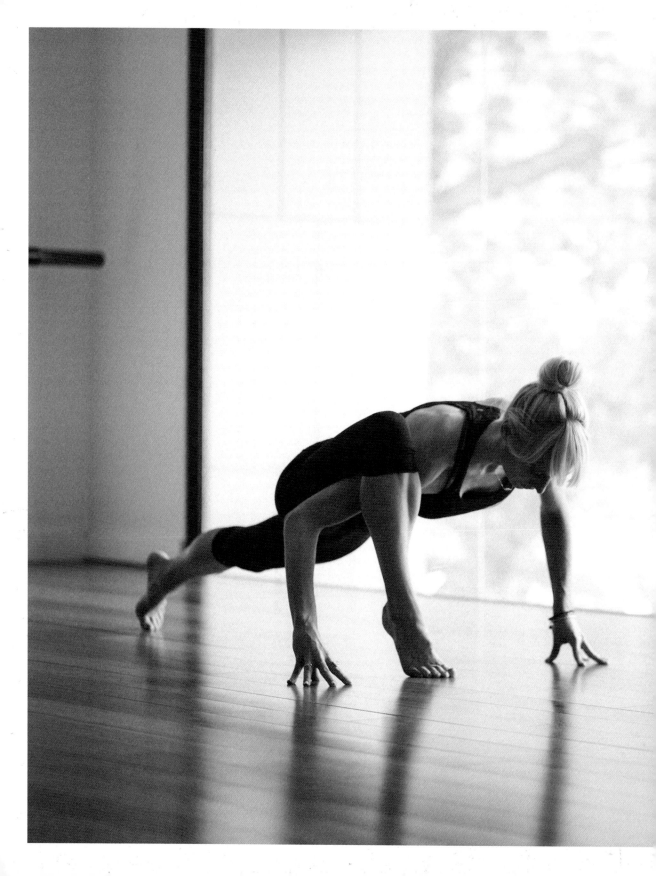

"Real life is right in front of you and I really want you to feel it, savour it and lean into it. Be you."

Does your phone have the upper hand?

How's your relationship with your phone?

Do you move from room to room in your own home with your phone in your hand?

Is checking it one of the first things you do in the morning (not to mention in the middle of the night)?

Do you freak out when you think you've lost it?

You could be addicted. Not joking. And in fact, many of us are.

And just like the chemistry of our chemicals, there's science that goes with that.[7,8]

Each time we get a like on Facebook or Instagram, it triggers a chemical response and releases dopamine – that feel-good hormone. The more comments and likes we get, the more we crave that feeling. It's no wonder you often find yourself checking your phone a thousand times a day – especially if you're feeling down. It's because you're after that feel-good dopamine hit.

Sometimes I even wonder if I own my iPhone or the iPhone owns me.

This tiny little thing that sits patiently in our handbag or pocket is pure genius. It does pretty much everything from paying bills to ordering food to wasting your time for at least an hour a day on

Instagram. It's no wonder that when you lose it (or think you've lost it, only to find that it was 'hiding' in your handbag) you freak the hell out.

Guilty as charged.

For me, part of that panic is the cost, time and effort associated with the thought of having to get a new one. And the other very big part of it is the thought of being isolated from the rest of the world until it's replaced.

But the thing is – the rest of the world is right in front of us, if only we could look up and around for long enough.

And you know, after the initial freak out, the moments spent phone free are rather liberating. Not being tethered to your phone has many upsides.

Fewer distractions.

A break for your nervous system.

Less comparison.

More real-time connection with the people in front of you.

Better for your posture and eyes (these are only two of the health benefits).

So maybe we need to look at our relationship with technology.

When you're with friends, how much of that time do you (and they) spend with phone in hand?

When you're with your partner, does one of you or both of you spend much of your quality time together on the phone? And how does that feel? Does it have an impact on the relationship? Do you feel closer for it or more distant?

Disconnected. Unrecognised. Separated.

These were words some of my friends responded with when I asked the above questions.

I think sitting together in silence is way more profound than filling the space with tech time.

Change the way you use your phone and watch your relationships change – including your relationship to self.

I really worry, in particular, about teenage girls who – before their feet have hit the ground of a morning – have already compared themselves with other girls on Facebook and Instagram. I want to shout out, hold them and tell them that the 'Gram is not real life.

Real life is right in front of you and I really want you to feel it, savour it and lean into it. Be you. Follow your heart and watch the world around you be magnetised to your energy. You're enough.

Right now could be the very moment you change your relationship to technology (clearly I'm using the phone as a scapegoat because it's the one most of us can relate to, but we also spend a lot of time on iPads, e-book readers, laptops, gaming consoles… and all the rest).

Just as alcohol was produced to be savoured and enjoyed, so too was the phone. It has a use and much purpose in our modern society. We can use it to stay connected to one another, including friends and family overseas, when it used to take very slow snail-mail to communicate with them. We can promote our businesses. We can make a difference to the world around us just with that tiny device. The phone has been a game changer in so many ways. But, just as we can binge on alcohol, we can over-use the phone.

What we can do with technology and, particularly, social media, is actually really exciting.

How awesome is it that we have this platform to project from? We can amplify our voices and be heard in a way possible in no other time. Women, especially, have a great opportunity to voice concerns and send their very much-needed messages out into the world. This is becoming more and more relevant.

So how about the next time you post something or make a comment, take notice. Is it coming from a place of ego (look at me and how fabulous my life is), or does it come from the heart?

Here's how I handle my iPhone cravings:

I set aside certain times during the day to look at it.

At night I have my iPhone on airplane mode so that I can still use it as an alarm but have no midnight distractions.

In the morning, it stays on airplane until after I've meditated.

In the evening I won't look at social media or emails during the two hours prior to bed. And this makes a huge difference to my quality of sleep.

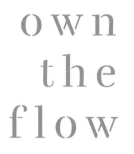

own the flow

DIGITAL DETOX

Choose one day a week to spend eight awake hours where you don't look at your phone or use it to do anything except make or answer calls.

At first you may find yourself doing the old 'phantom' move: without thinking, checking your bag or looking by your side for the phone that you've put out of sight.

Or you may notice the urge to check it every five minutes to see if someone's texted or liked a post. Don't look.

You won't regret this one.

Phone etiquette for the conscious yogi

In conversation: When distracted by your best friend (your phone), you're missing key signals from the person you're in conversation with. Put your phone away or if you put it on the table, lay it face down. You won't miss a thing and you'll create an opportunity to truly connect.

At meal times: Whether you're with another or hanging solo, put your phone away. Out of sight, out of mind. Not only will you experience some peace and quiet, and let your nervous system settle, but just as important, you'll give your digestion a better chance of working efficiently as you pay attention to your meal.

At bedtime: I keep my phone next to me to use as an alarm, but I power down two hours before bed, meaning there is no social engagement, texts or calls. And as I'm crawling into bed my phone goes onto airplane mode so there are no distractions, and less temptation to look on the way back from a midnight wee break.

Satsanga

Born out on sacrifice and built on love,
loyalty and honour

There's a word I learnt early on in my development as a yogi: satsanga.

This Sanskrit word means to associate with or be in the company of true people; it's often used to describe a group or a feeling.

I felt the meaning of it at the Dharma Shala, where I first practised yoga and later taught. I felt it when I ventured to India to do my first yoga teacher training, and where Satsanga was the name of the retreat I stayed at. I realise now, though, that way before I was introduced to yoga, I felt satsanga.

For a girl growing up in the country, it was considered snobbery if you did not look someone in the eye and say hello as you walked by. And it was drilled into me by my mother that I should always use someone's name. For a painfully shy little girl, this was hard, but I'm grateful to my mother for the moral and ethical upbringing I was given, which encouraged me to consider, care for and respect the people in the community around me.

I've been fortunate to have the support of community much of my life.

At the age of eleven, I was sent to boarding school. And before you assume my parents were wicked and mean, hold up. Boarding school was one of the best things to happen to me.

I was beyond excited to go. My older sister, Gina, was already there and I couldn't wait to be surrounded by all these girls, after feeling quite isolated on our apple farm just outside of Batlow. My primary school had a grand total of 40 pupils and in my year, at one stage, there were just six of us.

My hard-working parents, a nurse and an apple farmer, weren't exactly rolling in cash and so the decision to send us away, where they were confident we'd have a better education and more opportunity, was huge. And there's not a day that goes by when I reflect on my boarding school days that I'm not grateful for their sacrifices.

Thank you, Mum and Dad.

Although the number of people in my year jumped to 60 at boarding school, it was still small enough to know everyone in my year and to form incredibly close relationships with a great cluster of girls across several of the grades over the six years I was there.

There's something very special about the bonds you form in a live-in community like that.

Not only are the same girls there to say goodnight to, they're the same ones you wake to, share meals with, go on excursions with, study next to, play next to, chase boys next to, run amok with and generally go through all of those awkward teenage moments with.

They replace the constant support of parents. They become your shoulder to cry on, belly to laugh with and heck, as if by some energetic phenomenon (because it is), menstruation becomes in-sync too.

As many new friends as I may make today, there's nothing quite like the bond I formed with these girls. I may not see them as often as I'd like but when I do it's as if I still feel their essence: I know what's in their bones and they know what's in mine.

That experience of boarding school still goes down as one of my most cherished.

I learnt to share, contribute and consider others in a unique way. When you're literally living right next to the same girls for seven years, there's no other choice. And we had a damn good time.

After school I lived on campus at Macquarie University where I became a part of another community. Then later, when my business partner, Ben Lucas, and I opened Flow Athletic, this became my current and most relevant community to date.

Even before we opened the doors to the studio, we would sit and talk in our make-shift office – a table at Depot, a café in North Bondi – about the kind of community we wanted to bring into Flow Athletic. This was always clear for the two of us – and we didn't even have a business yet. We wanted to create a space for people to feel a part of something. Never did we just want to be a 'gym'. I was always adamant about maintaining the magic and tradition of yoga in this 'Yoga and Fitness' experience. And we wanted the benefits of satsanga, yoga philosophy and tradition to make their way into the strength and fitness rooms.

Today, one of the things that Ben and I are most proud of is that when members (or 'Flow Athletes') walk up the stairs, they feel a part of something. Yes, the classes are great, and our teachers are world class, but the real game changer is the relationships the members have with each other, and the people who work there.

We socialise together, train and practise together and we know that when we walk up the stairs to the studio, there are people there who care.

own
the
flow

LEANING INTO YOUR TRIBE

So, where do you seek your satsanga?
Where do you feel most a part of
a community?

Is it school? Uni? Mothers' group?
Your local gym or yoga studio?

Ask yourself: 'What can I do to feel a part
of that tribe? And how can I get involved
and contribute?'

It's incredible what comes from feeling
that you are part of something – a
community where individual souls
come together to co-create and make
a difference.

They say that if we want to feel good, we
do something for ourselves. And if we
want to feel fulfilled, we do something
for someone else.

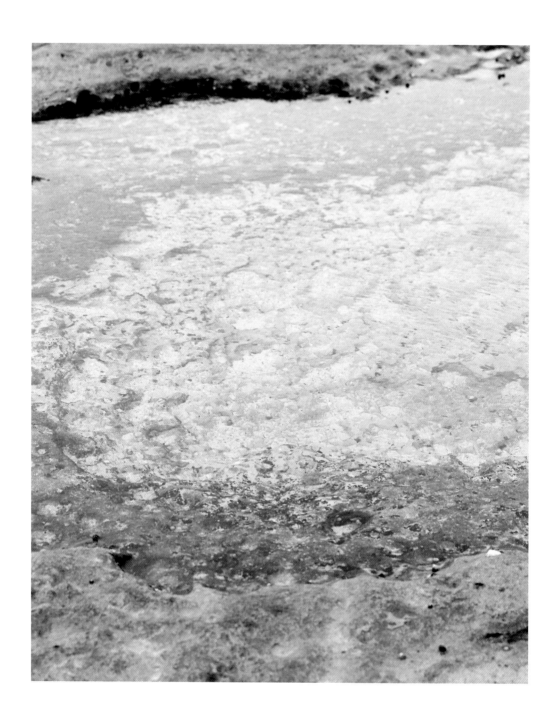

"A friend is someone who knows all about you and still loves you."

Elbert Hubbard, American artist and philosopher, 1856–1915

Circle of influence

Let's get real about who you're spending time with.

There's a theory that we're the average of the five people we spend the most time with.

How much truth there is behind that, I don't know. But it's an excellent conversation starter and self-enquiry activator. What do you think?

Personally, I think there's some truth to it. In light of my wish to be myself and live courageously, I want to surround myself with people who lift me up, challenge me and show me big, big love. I want to have a mix of people who are all mindfully making a difference to the world around them in their own significant ways.

I used to think it was important to have a huge network of friends – partly because I'm a chronic people pleaser and partly because I thought the more people I knew and connected with, the further I'd get in life. It's not what you know, it's who you know, right? Well... to a certain degree.

If we're intent on making those deep-down authentic connections, spreading your time and energy across 20 close friends is way more challenging (and exhausting) that spreading your time and love across a few really close ones, right?

As I mature, this is becoming more apparent to me.

One of my biggest lessons in the burn-out was re-prioritising both my joy and who really mattered in my life.

As we opened the business, to get people in the door, we hired a public relations company that did a smashing job. The company organised great yoga-based events and I became known, very quickly, as the face of the business. During this time I made a lot of 'influencer' friends. Influencers, in the PR world, are people who have a huge social media following and thus are viewed as having an influence over the decisions of their peers and audiences.

Did I have a lot in common with them? Not always. Sometimes, though, a lot. I'm lucky to still call a few of them very close friends. Perhaps the most 'in common' thing we all had was that we were on a mission to build our social empires – to build our businesses, or to gain more ambassador roles, which equated to dollars. And perhaps, for a few of us, it just fed our addiction to being 'liked'. It's not to say that each of them wasn't a genuine person when they went home to their loved ones – the ones they had really deep bonds with; it just meant that other relationships lacked depth.

This all became apparent during and after my burn-out. The friends that stood up and told me to pull my head in, to look after myself, and to remember what was really important were those high-school friends, plus a few other new friends who have become just as close.

These are the ones who really care. They each have their own way of showing it, but they each care. And I've really learnt to value that.

Sometimes it's important to look at our friendships more closely. Beyond those dear, close friends, many of us have other friends who have been around for a while. Perhaps they are other people you know from your school days; perhaps from an earlier job, which was the only thing you had in common. Perhaps you've stayed friends out of a sense of loyalty, but when you really look at it, you might realise that neither of you is serving the relationship in any way. Or perhaps just one of you is.

I want to say here that I don't think we should just start cutting friends straight away. Some relationships can be saved. It just takes some adjusting and shifting of the tone of your connection. For example, if you have a friend who spends your time together moaning about how hard done by she is, you could be the shining light in the relationship and point out all the good and great things in her life and all the opportunities she has in front of her – because they always exist. Sometimes we just can't see them until someone points them out.

And here's a big one. Are you in a long-time friendship with someone who bitches a lot? You may even join in on the bitching because that's what people do when they fear a lack of connection or what they say doesn't matter – they bitch. The first step is to notice that you have that kind of a relationship. Then if you care enough to save it, make the effort to change the tone of your conversations and direct things back to more positive commentary.

Or maybe you're involved in highly toxic friendships where the relationship thrives on getting wasted. What happens to the conversation and connection when you don't drink?

So, how's your circle? How do you make them feel? And how do you feel around them?

Could you shift the nature of the way you connect?

Swap gossip for conversations around growth.

Start swapping wines for walks – or at least a walk and then a wine!

And if the relationship still feels more toxic than terrific, perhaps it's time to let go.

own
the
flow

YOUR CIRCLE

Write down the names of the five people you spend the most time with.

Next to each person's name write the reasons why you love this person and how they make you *feel*.

mantra | cool. calm. connected.

Use this moving meditation to honour that very ancient philosophy that
we are all, in some way, divinely connected; that we're made up of the
same stuff as the stars and the trees and the wind and the ocean.

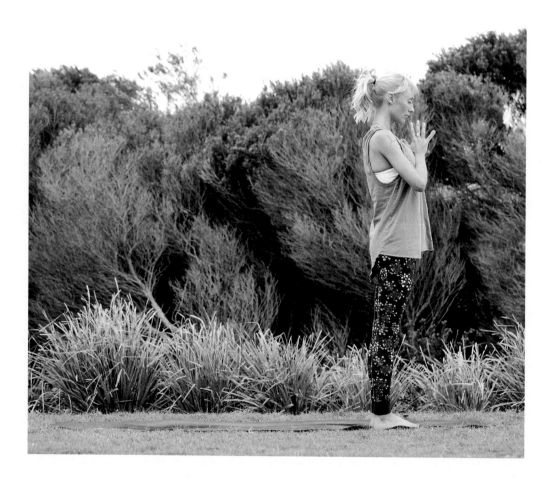

2. 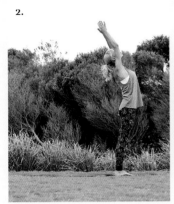 3. 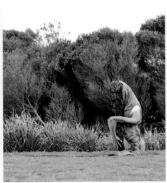 4.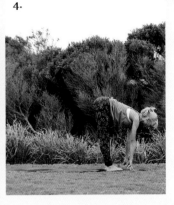

On the first round for each side (left and right as instructed below) stay in each posture for five breaths each, and then for each flow after that just one breath per movement. I suggest you take at least three rounds but on days when you have more energy, practise five to 10 times. But move slowly and remember to silently repeat your mantra: 'Cool. Calm. Connected.'

1 Anjali Mudra
Stand at the top of your mat checking that your feet are around hip distance apart. Take a moment to close your eyes and feel your feet firmly planted in this very moment, on the earth. Take your palms to face up with a bend in your elbows and repeat the mantra to yourself silently three times.

Bring your hands together at the heart and bow head to heart for a few moments. Affirm to yourself that you're exactly where you're meant to be.

2 Keeping the palms together, inhale and lift them up above your head (gazing up if it feels OK on the neck). As you ground down into your feet, keep the legs relatively active. You may even lift the chest up and back a little to create a tiny back bend. Go as far with this as feels good.

3 Fold Forward
As you exhale, take your arms out to the side to 'swan dive' forward and take your hands behind the calves or ankles, bending your knees as much as you need to if there is any strain in the lower back.

4 Half Lift
Inhale and lift your chest, taking hands to shins or finger tips to ground (if your hamstrings are tight, take hands to shins). Keep the back of your neck long while easing your chest forward.

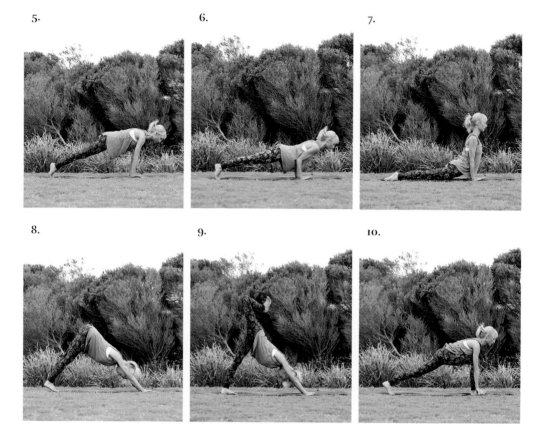

5.   6.   7.

8.   9.   10.

5 High Plank

As you exhale step both feet back into a plank position, with your wrists directly under your shoulders. Feel a long sloping line from head to heels. Your core supports this whole posture so draw your lower abdominal muscles and side waist in. Lightly energise the legs so you can feel the knee caps lift. Ease your collar bones forward, keeping the back of the neck long; there is still a gaze slightly forward, more with the eyes than the head.

6 Chaturanga

On an exhalation, while maintaining your plank form, tip forwards into the toes like you're peeking over the front of the mat, then bend your elbows to come down halfway. Check wrists and elbows are stacked and the elbows are close into the ribs.

7 Upward-Facing Dog

On your next inhalation, point the toes back (you may need to roll over them) to ease your chest forwards a little and then up. The tops of your feet are now pressing down into the Earth. Press down with the hands, allowing you to broaden the collar bones and ease the chest forward. Feel as though the back of your

II.

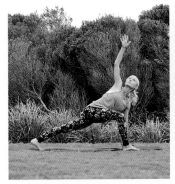

I2.

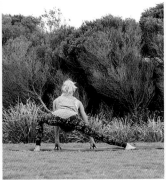

I3.

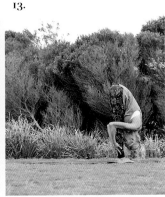

heart is easing forwards to the front of the heart.

8 Downward dog

On an exhalation, drawing on strength from your core, lift your hips up and back to arrive in downward dog. With hands shoulder distance apart and feet hip distance apart, ground the hands firmly (as if you could plunge them down and forwards into the Earth). If you are rounding through the spine or the hamstrings feel particularly tight, bend the knees as much as you need. Otherwise press your heels towards the earth. Wrap the outer edges of the upper arms in towards

each other and allow the neck to hang freely from the shoulders. Breathe and repeat your mantra.

9 Three-Legged Dog (with hip yawn)

On an inhalation, raise the right leg up and back behind you, at first keeping the hips square. On an exhalation bend your right knee and 'roll' the right hip open towards the side or sky (but ensure shoulders stay square to ground so that you're not just dropping into the left shoulder). On an inhalation square the hips again and step the right foot through between the hands to land in...

10 Lunge (right foot forward) Line up right ankle and knee and press firmly back into the left heel. Imagine you have a beach ball under the left leg which ensures that the left leg is supportive and active.

11 Lunging Twist

Maintain this strength and a sense of 'groundedness' in the legs and feet. Inhale your right arm out to the side and up. On the exhalation draw the navel gently into the spine to get the powerful detoxification magic of a twist. Stay a few breaths before...

12 Skandasana

On an exhalation, look down from your twist

and begin to turn the whole body to the left whilst pivoting on the feet. Place both hands on the ground in front of you. You will end up in a side lunge with the left knee and ankle stacked and the outer edge of your right foot fully grounded.

13 Step forward into Forward Fold

On an inhalation turn to face the front of the mat and step forward into half lift. Exhale to return to forward fold. Inhale to take your arms all the way out and up above the head and then exhale return to anjali mudra.

Repeat all 13 steps on the left side. Go slow.

Conscious connections

I crave deep connections.

I love being right in the middle of a delicious conversation where all parties involved are passionate, in their body and really listening to what the others have to say.

I love hanging with a mate on a park bench and feeling connected just through a few words but knowing that they are right there next to me, connected to the moment not only by the words but the space between them.

Confronting conversations really scare me sometimes, but I know that if I speak my truth and get my point across, while really listening to what the other person has to say, I will have grown just a little bit more by the end. I will have stepped out of my comfort zone and communicated from the heart. This too is a connection.

I love being there for a friend who has a broken heart: not intending to 'fix' things or make anything right, nor offer up advice to try to pull them out of their despair, but simply being there as a shoulder to cry on, truly listening.

These connections are soul expanding.

And when we think of conversations, we normally think of those with others, right? But the ones we have with ourselves, the inner dialogues, affect the ones we have with others. They can be critical to the health of our self-esteem and how we interact with the world around us.

I often encourage my students in class to explore their 'inner landscape'. By that I mean all the layers that make up their current state, physically, mentally and emotionally. It's about the overall tone of that inner space. When we stop talking and 'doing' for long enough, we can close our eyes and allow the inner gaze to light up. And if we look and listen for long enough, all kinds of thoughts, stories and narratives can come up – painful and beautiful alike. It's important to make space for the full range of thoughts to arise, negative and positive, because often they just need to be recognised. What we do with them is always our choice and the more conscious we become (which, by the way, is a daily practice) the more we can choose the thoughts that serve.

Outside voice and inside voice

How's your self-chat?

Did you know we have thousands of thoughts every single day - and sometimes as many as 60 per cent of them can be negative?[10]

Have you ever thought about how powerful the words you speak are?

So powerful, in fact, that if we use certain ones for long enough, they become our truths.

Let's look at positive affirmations.

'I am worthy of love and belonging.'

Apparently the jury is still out about how useful affirmations really are, although research suggests it can help in a range of situations, from academic achievement to self-control[11,12,13]. Personally, I think we have to start somewhere and if words help to get the ball rolling, then why not?

'I am worthy of love and belonging.' When repeated daily and frequently, the vibrations of these words will carve out new thought pathways. Soon enough, if you build enough awareness and resilience to act in alignment with this positivity, it can become your reality.

And P.S. You were always worthy of love and belonging, but perhaps somewhere along the way you decided that you weren't. You stopped 'affirming it' to yourself. And what happens when the universe keeps sending you gifts of love and belonging, and you reject them? It stops sending them until you change your attitude or affirmation. If we were the universe we'd probably do the same thing!

The same is true of negative affirmations. If you're constantly telling yourself 'I'm not good enough', you'll make choices that ensure you're proved right.

So... how's your self talk?

What are you telling yourself every day? What are the stories that you are repeating outwardly about yourself day after day?

Let's look at the two different kinds of chat.

Inside voices: The unfiltered conversations you have with yourself.

Outside voices: The chat you have with the people around you. The kind of chat that can really connect you to another human being.

Both types of chat are important, but we need to remember that the inner voice will eventually have an impact on the outer voice.

There are various types of outside voices.

Surface-value 'weather' or 'water cooler' chat: this is often just a space filler, but it can be useful in breaking the ice between people who don't know each other very well.

Business chat: the conversations that are logistical or useful, or help organise the lives we live.

Social and networking chat, in person and online.

And then my favourite: deep, profound and genuinely connected to your heart chat. It's a conversation of truth and when you're in it, time stands still. Chats like this lead to expansion and growth.

All of these can be influenced by the two main inside voices: trash talk (which comes from fear) and love talk.

Being mindful of the inner voice is the first step to mastering it.

Here's a sample of my inside voice from a typical morning a few years ago. I wrote a blog about it that day and I also share it in my online e-course, 'The Space Between'.

———

Seemingly fine, I wake up and stroll to the bathroom and here's what transpires:

Looks in mirror.

Oh wow. I look tired. How am I going to get rid of those bags under the eyes today? Maybe it's time for Botox. If only I had (insert name of friend who has seemingly flawless skin)'s genetics.

Looks down.

So bloated this morning. Fu*k. I'm having a fat day. What am I going to wear? I have that meeting in the city and I want to make a good impression but my whole wardrobe is stretchy pants. I really need to do a shop. All my clothes are tired and old... not like (insert various names and faces of fashionable friends) who make fashion look effortless and chic. Always. Starts brushing teeth.

Oh, crap, I didn't send the email about the thing last night and I've totally forgotten to brief the team on the other thing. I'm always letting people down. People must think I'm a flake. Actually – it's not my fault I'm a flake – I don't get enough sleep because I over-work.

But if I don't work hard people will think I'm lazy. I will be lazy. That's weak. No one ever does anything good in this world by being weak.

Pauses to wonder how long she's been brushing teeth and feels like her gums might fall out she's been brushing so ferociously.

———

And all this 'stinking thinking' takes place over about 10 seconds. Imagine the rest of the rubbish that goes on for the other 86,390 seconds of the day?

See how I go from one negative thought about myself to self-doubt, to comparison, to mean girl to victim and then blame in one fell swoop? And this is how I've started my day.

You can see why meditation is such an instrumental and productive part of your morning. Even if you do take the time to clean your teeth first – which I always do – you can return to your seated posture (or however you meditate) and let the already transpired inner dialogue settle and clear, to make way for the rest of your day.

The thing I learnt from writing about that experience is that in those first few moments of the day before I take my 'seated practice', it's relevant to catch the thoughts and be clear on their tone. Mornings are the perfect time to do this because generally the mind is a little clearer from slumber and our nervous system has rested.

After that morning, and writing the blog post about it, I had a Post-it note on the bathroom mirror for a few weeks. 'Mind the tone, KK,' it said. Even though that little piece of paper wilted and peeled off, its effects have lingered.

If the tone of the above chat sounds familiar, lean in. Listen up. Here's my rant that I hope hits you in just the right way.

Most of the stuff we tell ourselves is absolute bullsh*t.

Do you think I'm overweight? No – I'm not. And if I were – does that mean I'm not worthy of love and belonging? Nope.

Do I have the same youthful face as the 23-year-old I was comparing myself with? No. Because I'm not 23 anymore. Truth. And does that mean I'm not as worthy of love or belonging? No, we're all worthy. We're all enough. We all have everything we need to feel deeply connected and loving, to ourselves and others. The exterior changes, but the soul inside remains the same. And that's who we truly are.

It's our ego that tells us we're not enough.

The ego gets a pretty bad rap sometimes. But it's there to teach us, to enlighten us. It shows us contrast and calls upon our inner-most resilience in order to see truth.

The good news is that if you keep following a path of mindfulness and truth seeking, you'll have sweet victory over the ego, or at least call it on its bullsh*t and not act on it each and every time.

Rant over.

So, if you really are having the same thoughts as yesterday…

How's that working for you?

I know, because you are here, reading this book and these words, that you're up for a more vibe-high, self-actualised existence, today and every day.

It's just not possible to switch off our thoughts. And why would we want to? They're useful and they send us some damn good ideas sometimes.

All I'm suggesting is that we change the tone of the negative self-talk to one of positivity for more of the time.

Even the negative thoughts have a purpose. They push us, question us and keep us striving to be better humans. But if we linger in them for too long they become our reality.

Thoughts are based in love or fear. You get to choose. Only always.

Expansion versus contraction

Expansiveness is our natural state.

Think about the moments you've felt most at ease, most relaxed and most open: fluent and in flow with the people and places around you. When you felt most connected.

You were, most probably, in a state of 'expansion'. Perhaps you'd just been on a week-long retreat or a relaxing holiday. Perhaps you were falling in love, or were surrounded by people who made you feel loved and who you loved in return.

Perhaps you're in that state right now.

And then remember a time when you felt closed and contracted – 'out of flow'.

You didn't want to socialise or speak with people. You distrusted, tried to control the people and situations around you and generally had a fairly poor outlook on life. Perhaps this was triggered in response to an argument with your love or because you were going through some stage of change that scared you.

Perhaps you're in that state right now.

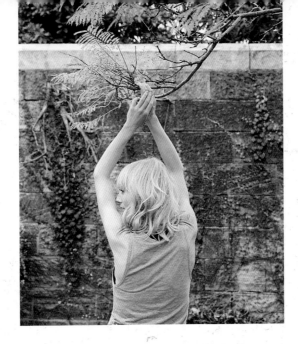

Quite often our state is influenced by triggers. Some trigger pleasure and some pain. How long we wade or float in either state is up to us.

A trigger is a full body (mental and physical) reaction to something that is happening in the present but that jogs a memory. From this past experience, we've formed behaviours, sometimes life-long ones, that kick in when a trigger gets us.

For example, my older sister, Gina, is bossy. She knows this. We (my family and I) know this. It's part of why we love her. And she's been bossing me, as older siblings do so well, my whole life.

Now that we are both adults, she still does it. And even though we laugh and joke it off, when she orders me to do something (these days she disguises it as a request, but it is sugar-coated with 'boss'), I still revert to the four-year-old who obeys at her every demand.

Her words trigger me. They shift me into a pattern of 'doing' that I developed in childhood. I feel contracted and on edge. I feel the 'doing' in my nervous system and I end up acting out the pattern until I realise what's going on.

Here's another example that I think you might relate to.

You've had your heart broken early on in your teenage or early adult years by a lover and it hurt. So bad. It hit you right in your heart and for some time thereafter, you closed it. If you had really leaned in at the time you would probably have become aware of this energetic contraction.

Over time, your heart moves on and you eventually open again. Until you're with another lover. You're only a few months into the relationship, and your heart feels as though it might explode it's so open. And then one day, he or she does something to remind you of that former lover who hurt you. They say something that triggers a response in you and, before you can say, 'over-red-rover', your heart is closed tight. You're once again in that state of contraction.

In reality, the current lover has only uttered some words. He or she is not even thinking about breaking up with you. And they quite understandably have no idea what's going on. Why, all of a sudden, have you closed yourself off, they wonder. They can feel the distance, the wall, and this only creates more separation between the two of you. This can go on for some time unless you have an open dialogue about how each of you are really feeling. Sometimes that happens eventually, but sometimes it doesn't.

The sooner we can be aware of these triggers and their response, the sooner we can learn to let go.

own
the
flow

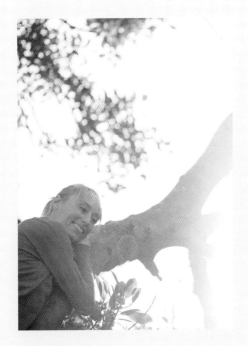

EXPANSION V CONTRACTION

At any point in your day, whether you're
being triggered or not, take your awareness
to your heart and ask:

'Am I in a state of expansion or
contraction?'

Does the heart feel rigid, hard or closed?
Perhaps the chest area feels tight.

Or does it feel soft, malleable and open.
Perhaps the chest area feels relaxed.

At first, the answer might take some time
to come, but the more you practise, the
easier it gets and can have a profound
effect on your state.

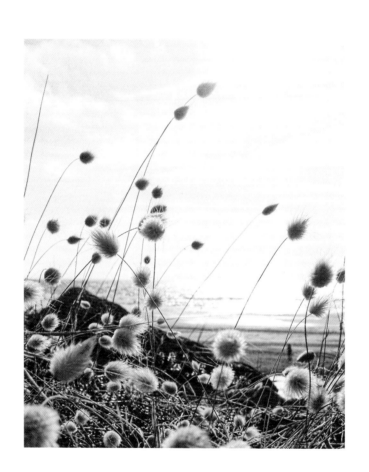

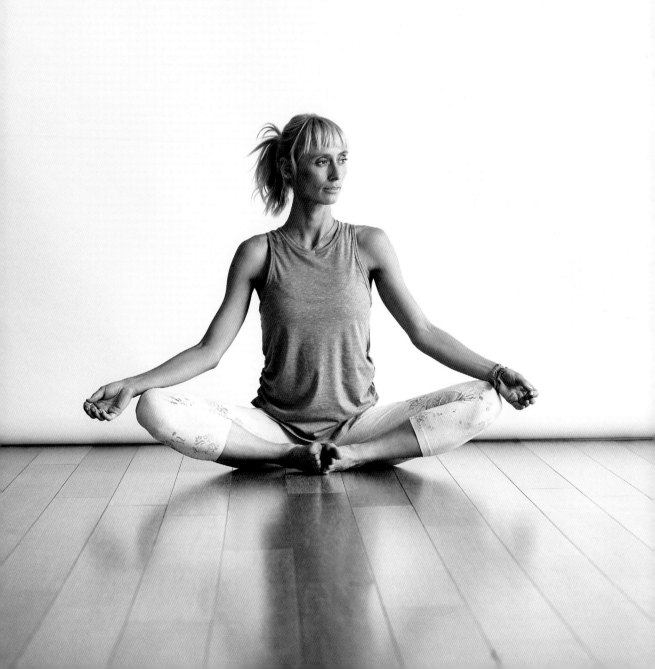

PHILOSOPHY 101.
Samskaras

I've been teaching yoga for more than a decade now and observing
my students has taught me things too. I've watched some of the
repetitive behaviours students exhibit during yoga class that
I suspect originated long before they stepped onto the mat.
And I'm aware of the ones that play out on the mat for me, too.

For example, I tend to 'over-do', over-push and over-strive. I've been
called an over-achiever and it's probably the reason I burnt out and
why I have written this book. It's not necessarily a bad thing. In fact,
it's contributed to the success I've had as a young athlete and
business woman.

It becomes a problem, and detrimental to my health, however, when
I don't take time out, give myself some 'space between' or recover
properly. Striving has never been a crime. It's pushing too hard that
lands me in trouble.

I know this tendency is playing out on the mat when I feel obliged to
do every single posture (especially the most advanced) offered up by
the teacher. There are days when my energy is lower and I know the
more 'advanced' yogi in me would rest instead of revving up to the
challenge. That's what an advanced yogi does: they listen to their
body. And sometimes the strongest thing I'll do is rest. But when
I choose negative behaviour patterns and ego over listening to the
body, all the sweetness leaves the practice.

Pushing too hard – what I call over-striving, whether it happens on
the mat or off the mat – is born from ego. It took me a good year of
practising to really notice this habit and make the parallel.

Whatever we practise on the mat, we practise off the mat.

The yoga studio is simply the arena in which we can witness our deeply ingrained habits in all their glory. According to yogic philosophy, we're born with a karmic inheritance of mental and emotional patterns — known as samskaras — through which we cycle over and over again during our lives.

The word samskara comes from the Sanskrit sam (complete or joined together) and kara (action, cause or doing). In addition to being generalised patterns, samskaras are individual impressions, ideas, or actions; taken together, our samskaras make up our conditioning, or how we see and react to the world.

Repeating samskaras reinforces them, creating deep grooves that are challenging to resist.

Samskaras can have a profoundly positive effect on our own wellbeing as well as those of others. Look to the workings of humanitarians who can't help but 'give' so that others have better lives.

These patterns can also have a negative effect on our mental health and wellbeing: think of the harmful self-beliefs that tell us we're not enough, that we need to be prettier, thinner, more successful, more recognised.

But here's the good news. Practising our yoga on and off the mat can help break the patterns. It can help us be conscious of what's going on and notice the triggers as they arise.

We can, moment by moment, by practising mindfulness, stay aware of our physical, emotional and psychological responses. We can acknowledge them as they happen and gently let them go. We can feel what we feel and release it energetically.

In other words, there are always going to be things that trigger us but we can, with practice, learn not to react to them.

And in that moment of deciding not to react in the same old way, some serious magic happens.

Instead of deepening those grooves and patterns, we become strong enough to 'change the track' and create new pathways.

Some of these grooves are deep and moving out of them is challenging — perhaps our biggest life's work. But breaking away from those old, instinctive reactions and creating more positive and healthy ones is truly liberating.

So what are some of your patterns?

What triggers you and what behaviour follows? If you observe yourself for a day or two, you'll notice your patterns. If you've got nothing going on and can't think of any, great, have some of mine! But most of us will find our triggers if we watch closely enough. Here are some examples to get things started:

Trigger: Someone gives you a compliment, but you feel unworthy.

Response/Behaviour: You laugh it off or change the subject.

Trigger: You jump on Instagram to see what's up and scroll through image after image of girls on sunny beaches in barely there bikinis or guys who are chiselled and chilled and seem to have it all figured out.

Response/Behaviour: With a knot in your chest you navigate your way to the fridge and numb out with a bowl of ice cream or a few bottles of beer.

Trigger: You partner gets home at 3am, a reminder of the behaviour of that guy who cheated on you a few years ago.

Response/Behaviour: Can't sleep. When he wakes up in the morning you're suspicious and untrusting and make it very known in a passive aggressive kind of way (which is the worst, ever, right!?).

The list goes on. And if you pay really close attention you'll notice that these triggers are everywhere. Absolutely everywhere. If they were visible, tangible things we'd literally be drowning in them.

But we don't have to be. We most definitely do not have to be slaves to the trigger.

This is why meditation and yoga are so incredibly powerful. They teach us to not sweat the small stuff; to practise patience in a way that allows us to step back from our triggers for long enough to see what's really going on in our bodies at the time.

This 'stepping back for long enough' brings us to another aspect of 'the space between': that gap between stimuli and response.

That pause can be profoundly potent, and hugely productive.

The pause isn't just about waiting. It's to be leaned into. Bravely.

You can use the RAIN technique again for dealing with samskaras or patterns — try the Own the Flow on the following pages.

own
the
flow

RAIN FOR TRIGGERS

RAIN, which I mentioned before in Chapter 2, is a four-step technique used in mindfulness to observe a situation. Where once we may have gone on auto-pilot and snapped straight into reactive mode, RAIN (Recognise, Allow, Investigate, Nurture) helps to us to see, soften and surrender in a way that is super strong. It may just be one of the most useful skills you'll acquire.

Recognise that we've been triggered.

Allow the emotion or feeling that comes with it to 'be'. In other words – make space for it. We could also call this step accept, because the moment you resist something, the energy around it gets stronger. Allowing, on the other hand, softens. Just like people, sometimes emotions just need to be heard.

Investigate the emotion and where you 'feel' it in the body. It can often show up as tension in the abdomen or shoulders, or perhaps you clench your jaw, or tap or fidget.

Nurture means to lean into the felt experience. Don't think there's something wrong about what you feel; don't go numb. Stay. Use the 90-second rule. I've also heard this step called Non-Attachment, asking us not to take it personally, to realise that how we're feeling is universal. What you feel, others feel, and it's all your body's attempt to protect you. Here is where can say 'Thanks jealousy (or anger or regret or whatever emotion you are feeling), but I don't need you right now'.

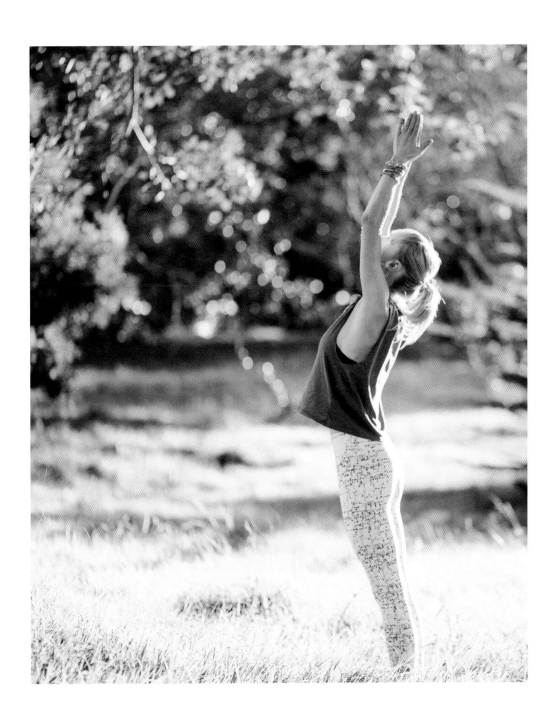

Yogi 3

MICHAEL TREMBATH

Michael is the real deal. He's been on a rich spiritual journey and has mountains of wisdom acquired from his guru and his travels through spiritual places such as India. He also has a natural ability to lean in and 'feel' more than the average human dares to. It's a gift that I believe we all have, but don't often tap into.

My relationship with him is multi-faceted.

I consider him a mentor, spiritual coach, guide, cheerleader, energetic healer and, most of all, dear friend.

There is a deep sense of love within and pouring forth from this man's whole being that I've never felt before. And it's a result of being deeply connected (that word again). He is empathetic and understanding. He can lean into your own energy and emotions in a way that makes you realise that we're all connected. I feel what you feel and what we do to one we do to all.

The way his sessions work is hard to describe. Generally, you start with a little chat while he reads your pulse. His method of work is Samvahan, an ancient Indian vibrational healing technique. The reading of the pulse is to get a sense of how your organs are working and whether there are any imbalances he can work on. You then lie on a massage table and he proceeds to move energy around your body. He can sense blockages and move them to make your energy more at harmony and ease. Sometimes we talk through the session and that helps to highlight blockages for which he will give me practical energetic visualisations or exercises to move the energy. Sometimes we don't talk at all. We go with the flow.

Besides his gifts as a healer and the fact that he balances me so well, I love his outlook on life. He's playful and never takes things too seriously; he never labels anything as good or bad but rather accepts it is. He reminds me that everything in life has a cycle and changes. Everything passes. He deeply cares and loves. When you speak, he is in his body and really listens, without the need to get a point across or even speak back – he's just 'right there'. He's humble and holds himself with integrity. I think perhaps he's the kindest man I know. And I love him so much.

He is one of the most connected individuals I know. To do what he does takes that. If he's not 'tapped' into his own mental, physical and energetic self, he can't tap into and heal anyone else. Connection is his priority.

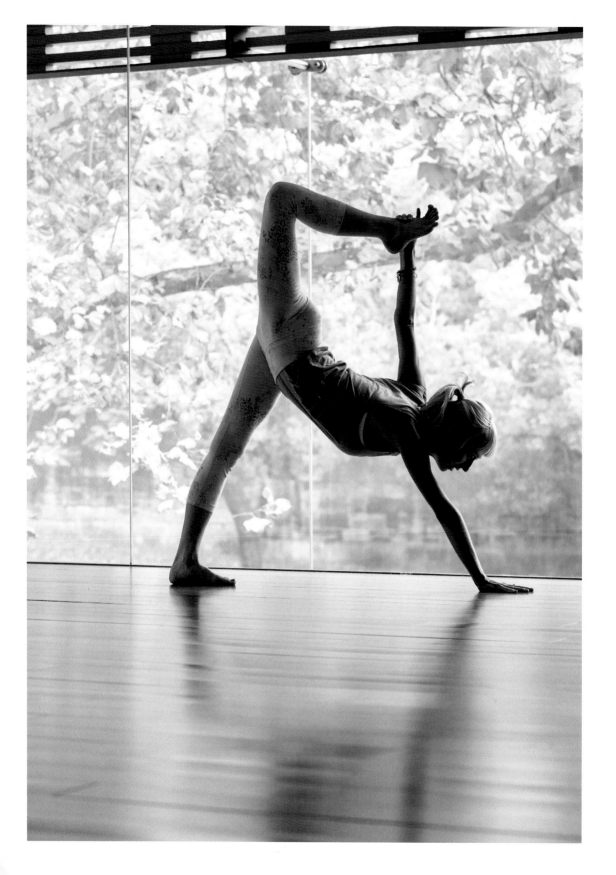

own
the
flow

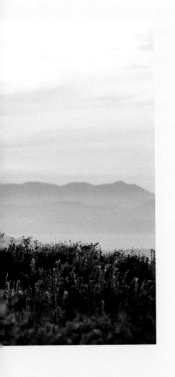

MOVING THE ENERGY

This one is inspired largely by my friend and mentor Michael Trembath.

When you find yourself in 'reactive mode' or triggered by something, as hard as it can be sometimes, take a few moments to close your eyes (you could be standing, seated or lying) and locate where you feel the emotion in your body.

Give it a colour and possibly a texture. Don't over-think it – go with the colour and texture that comes up first.

Stay with the sensation of it and after being with it for a minute or so, watch the colour and texture start to move from that place in the body and flow down to the feet and out into the Earth.

The key is to move the energy. When energy gets stuck we end up with ailments, fatigue and disease.

Moving it creates flow and harmony in the body. In other words, it's OK to have the emotion come up, but it's important for our health to move it so that it doesn't metastasise or get stuck.

The art of conversation

I used to meet up with a friend for coffee. I wouldn't say we were close but definitely friendly enough to catch up every couple of months and share stories on our new businesses and their developments.

He was athletic, charismatic and carried himself with confidence.

When he spoke, he was engaging, funny and magnetic. I found myself captivated and often on the edge of my seat waiting for the punchline in his clever analogies and stories. However, I would often leave the setting of our catch-ups somewhat deflated. And I didn't know why.

Until one day the penny dropped.

I had listened for a good hour of our 75-minute lunch date to his charming-as-ever stories and updates on the development of his latest project. I congratulated him on his ballsy approach to what seemed like a risky endeavour and then started to talk about one of my own projects.

At Flow Athletic, we were just starting to expand our Flow After Dark Silent Disco yoga to a much larger scale with an upcoming event at Sydney's Hordern Pavilion. We were taking it next level! At the previous event we'd had 200 and this time we were aiming for 1500. I was so excited and nervous about it that I found myself lost in an animated rave about it. But my excitement wasn't met. I noticed my friend gazing over my shoulder at someone behind me. Then his eyes darted to the door of the cafe as a good-looking girl walked in.

And in that moment I realised why I had felt deflated all those times.

When it was time for me to share my experiences, my friend lost interest, and became disengaged and distracted. And there was a very definite energetic wall that came up.

And it made me realise that conversation has to be two-way. It's one thing to engage someone in chat — anyone who's quite charismatic is great at this. But if you're not taking turns, if you're not listening, you may as well be having a conversation with a brick wall, right?

I'm still friends with this charismatic human and actually ended up giving him this feedback plus asking for his permission to tell this story. And we're all good. He had no idea he was doing it and as a result of the conversation, we're now much tighter.

It also made me question whether there were people that I did the same thing to. Was there anyone I didn't give my full attention to in our conversations?

And the answer was yes.

Sometimes when I am rushed or busy, my mind is elsewhere, and I don't quite 'keep up' in the conversation. I don't pay attention. I can miss important cues or information within what someone may be telling me.

Turns out my friend's lesson was also mine.

So how do you think you are in the art of conversation?

Are you a great listener but find it hard to share? Or do you share like a champion but find it hard to listen?

I'm going to take a stab in the dark and say most of us, even if we are good listeners, could probably fine tune our listening skills and become more grounded in the way we show up for others.

Deep listening

I've made a few trips to Uluru in the centre of Australia. Anyone who's been there will likely relate to my feelings about the magnetic energy surrounding the rock, the surreal size of this natural wonder and sheer beauty of such a random formation in the middle of nowhere.

On one such trip, co-leading a retreat with Michael Trembath, there was a moment – just as the sun went down – where the group we were with couldn't help but be pulled into silence. It was as if, in deep reverence for both the rock and the sun that had been beating down on it all day, the visitors were lulled into stillness – the kind that begs to be listened to.

And it got me thinking.

When you're grounded and solid in yourself, like a rock, it's magnetic.

Uluru sits in stillness, grounded some several kilometres below (no one really knows how far down it goes). It can't help but have presence.

Out in nature, all you can hear is just that – birds, wind… flies. The moment. If you listen for long enough, you can really connect with the energy below you. The same goes for listening in conversations.

Listening pulls talking. Listening pulls truths.

Be with someone in conversation for long enough, without talking too much or interrupting, and that person will reveal truths. They will feel comfortable to bare their soul and feel fully heard. And isn't that one of the greatest gifts you can give someone?

own
the
flow

GIVING AND RECEIVING
IN CONVERSATION

I often include this exercise in my teacher training sessions, and find it's effective in building conscious conversation.

Next time you're communicating with someone try these two exercises.

First, get grounded. Take a few deep breaths and send your awareness to your legs and feet – a reminder that you're planted right here and now.

Then:

When talking: *Place one hand onto your abdomen (as a reminder to connect with your breath) and speak mindfully. Notice your tone of conversation. (Is it trash talk about someone? Does it align with your values? Are the words coming from your highest self? Do you mean it?)*

If you notice yourself talking too much, talking for the sake of it or trash talking and gossiping – how about not? How about holding back and focusing on the breath. No words are often way more powerful, not to mention energy saving. Try it. At first you may feel as if you're not contributing, because you've gotten into such a habit of over-talking. You'll find, though, after some practice, that holding back is fuelled with integrity, power and strength.

When listening: *Place one hand onto your abdomen (as a reminder to connect with your breath) and listen mindfully.*

Don't interrupt the other person. If there is a gap for you to add something of relevance, take a deep breath first then speak.

Remember... listening pulls truth.

CHAPTER 4

Devotion

being of service

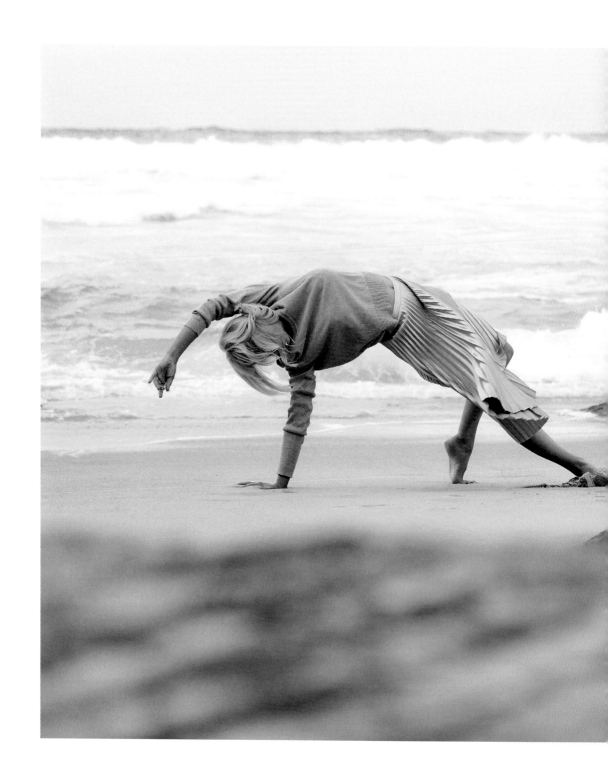

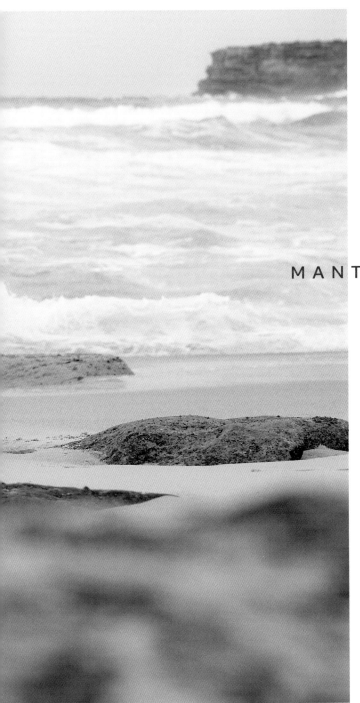

MANTRA:

GRACE

"The sun never says to the earth, 'You owe me'. Look what happens with a love like that. It lights the whole sky."

Hāfiz, Persian poet, 1325–1390

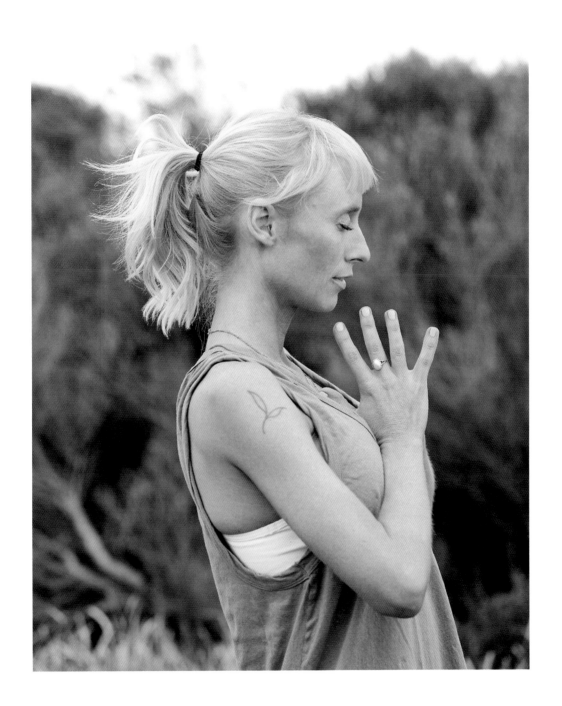

What we give, we get back. *Only always.*

It's a universal law. A universal truth and a guiding principle for anyone striving to live a purpose-FULL, productive and potent life.

Devotion, at its very essence, is being in service to something other than self.

Some of us are devoted to Gods or Goddesses. Some devote themselves to a worldly cause while others are devoted to the tiny humans they've brought into this world. I'm surrounded by people who devote their life to a career that lights them up and makes them feel connected and fully alive.

And when we're really living this devotion, we realise that even though the effort is being made in order to give to something or someone 'else', there's no separation between you and that thing you're giving service to. You and that thing become one.

In giving to other – you're giving to self.

This theory can't simply be 'understood' intellectually. It must be fully felt. Fully experienced. And the only way to do that is through giving.

So what are you devoted to?

Diversification in devotion is required to have a global community that truly cares – not only for one another, but for every corner of the planet.

It's as though we each have a unique calling; and those callings are perfectly splattered and scattered among the populations. Everyone has a role to fulfil in the order of the world. And here's the thing – when you find that thing that you're devoted to (and I think, by the way, it's OK to change your mind... multiple times) you light up. People notice because it's magnetic, inspiring and totally on point.

We know we're living 'on purpose' when through acts of service, we feel so damn good.

I'll never forget one afternoon during my university years. I was hanging out with an old school friend, Lucy, also one of my best mates. Always quite 'spiritual' and connected to God when we were moving through our teenage years, she'd recently found a modality called NLP, or Neuro Linguistic Programming.

She started using some of the techniques on me. I was in awe. Yes, partly because this was some of that deep work that I was yearning to get into myself but hadn't quite found, but it was more than that. It was the way she lit up when she talked about it. The promise of this technique's ability to transform lives and reframe mindsets seemed really promising. And whether or not I believed that didn't matter, because Lucy's dedication to the learning process she was going through was red hot. I so clearly remember her saying 'I'm going to dedicate my life to this'. And I believed her. There wasn't an inch of doubt. It was said with such conviction. I could tell that this was coming straight from her soul, through the heart and throat and out as an expression of devotion.

And to this day, she does. She's shifted away from some of the modalities but the theme and tone of what she's doing is bang on.

Why I remember that moment so clearly, I don't know. I knew I didn't want to pursue the exact same things, so perhaps there was part of me that yearned to know what my legacy would be. What was I going to dedicate my life to, and how could I be of service? I knew that was the whole point from quite an early age – which caused frustration because I hadn't worked out what that service was. It was a deep yearning with no obvious answer straight away. It took time.

I think it's frustrating for many young people, and often more mature people too, who are searching for that 'thing' that lights them up. As far as I can tell there's no intended time for you to come across this. But what I do know is that if you 'follow the charm' often and with enough courage, you'll find it. Time and time again.

We're in constant co-creation with the universe.

What we give to it – it gives back.

But if we spend our whole time playing the victim, wondering when it's 'our time' or hoarding all of our winnings, skills, talents and money, then that steady and even universal flow of life energy gets stuck. We cease to have things come back to us.

So again, how are you in service? And are you making it a priority?

Not just in what you do for a living but the everyday things. After all, how we do one thing is how we do all.

Is there a legacy you want to leave behind? What is it that you want your grandchildren and children, or other young people who matter to you, to say about you after you've left this life? Life's short. In some way or another we all know this. Just look at how the years rush by.

Grab life and decide. Start with the small things, such as the choices you make when you do your weekly shopping, the people you spend your time with and the media that you choose to buy and 'buy into'.

It all counts. Start now.

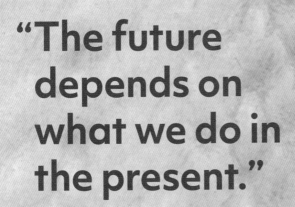

"The future depends on what we do in the present."

Mahatma Gandhi, Indian civil rights leader, 1869–1948

Giving and receiving

And the interconnection between them

The yogi understands that there is no separation between them and the universe: that every living being, thing, object and cause is intrinsically connected.

When one truly understands this, giving becomes not only fun but fulfilling. To be able to take your awareness from self to other can help you out of dumps of depression and mild cases of anxiety. You realise that there is more to life. There's a much bigger picture than the dramas that are playing out in your own head.

Yes, sometimes big stuff happens that we need to lean into and pay attention to, but for the most part we could diminish the drama, open our eyes to what's around us and realise that by helping others, we help self. It's a beautiful collaboration.

We can't really expect to give fully without also being able to receive. It's a two-way street. One without the other lacks lustre. The two combined are a potent recipe for manifesting what you want in life.

One of my favourite books is a tiny but terrific little read: *The Seven Spiritual Laws of Success* by Deepak Chopra. The laws are universal truths that can help us navigate life and understand it, in order to live in harmony with the things that seem out of our control.

One such law, The Law of Giving and Receiving, states that the two are different expressions of the same flow of energy in the universe. Since the universe is in a constant and dynamic exchange of energy, you need both the give and take to maintain a steady flow of abundance, love and anything else you want to manifest in your life.

We can consciously cultivate an environment for that flow to be abundant and flourish, although not without discipline and effort at times. It's rather easy, but totally energy zapping, to drop into a selfish state of take, take, take. To think only of one's self, especially when we're down, and to close ourselves off from those around us.

All human beings represent an opportunity to give. All people, situations and places are 'on purpose' and when we intentionally make space for them, magic happens. And giving doesn't always have to be at the cost of your back pocket or bank account. Giving could be wishing a stranger good fortune; silently blessing a friend who is going through something traumatic; dedicating your next surf, walk, yoga practice, meditation or the savouring of a meal to someone who needs the energy of that activity; or perhaps the biggest give of all – giving your time.

It's not about the money. It's what we put behind the act that counts.

Do you ever – or often – find yourself meaning to 'give' in some way, but then not following through? Too busy, not sure of how… it happens to us all. But intention without action is kind of useless. And, if repeated often, can make us feel rather shallow. There is a way past this – it just takes practise.

The thought to give starts at the heart, then the follow through comes from the solar plexus region, which yoga and energy anatomy says is the place in which our discipline, will power and confidence reside. Giving wholeheartedly is a beautiful co-creation between these two energetic centres of heart and solar plexus.

The Own The Flow that follows is a stunning visualisation that I love. It reminds me of how these two centres work together and helps cultivate an effortless flow between the two.

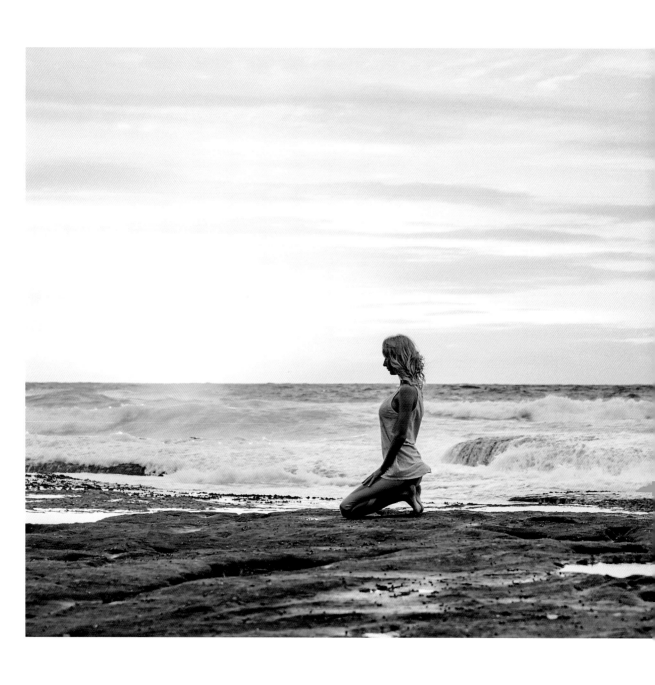

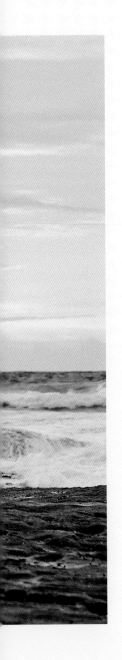

own
the
flow

INFINITY FLOW

Take five minutes to close your eyes
and get grounded. Silently repeat this
mantra three times: 'I cultivate the
flow of abundance effortlessly.'

Let your breath be relaxed and soft
and rest your awareness on your heart.
'Live' in your heart for a few moments,
watching it being breathed (expanding
and contracting) with the breath. Then
drop your awareness to the solar plexus
region and, again, watch it (or the
abdomen) being breathed.

Now begin to carve out a figure eight,
or infinity sign, that loops around the
top of the heart, down across the midline
of the body and under the solar plexus
then makes its way back up, across the
midline of the body and over the top of
the heart again.

It may take a few moments to find a flow
but when you do, maintain that gentle
awareness and ride its flow, whilst silently
repeating the mantra: 'I follow my heart's
natural intention to give and receive with
even flow.'

Karma Yoga – serving the world without expecting anything in return

How good does it feel to give?

The yogis have known this felt experience and call being of service 'Karma Yoga'.

I'll often begin leading yoga classes by asking students to dedicate their practice to something or someone if it feels right. In this, we're not giving anything physical, but we are devoting our practice to something other than self. And that accounts for a lot.

How we give, and the energy behind it, says a lot about our intention.

Christmas, birthdays, special occasions, just-for-the-sake-of-it...

We all know the difference between giving out of obligation (which is a horrible reason to give, right?) and giving with our whole heart.

Giving out of obligation feels pushed, gritty and, potentially, layered with bitterness. I think most of us can relate to that feeling of being invited to a distant friend's birthday party (that you just don't want to go to anyway) and then, on top of that reluctance, having to search for and spend money on a present. All for someone you're not that into. It just feels like a waste, right?

DEVOTION

Giving out of obligation will be noticed. If it feels inauthentic to give, that same sense of inauthenticity is felt on the other end, by the receiver, too.

Contrast this, then, to giving with your whole heart.

Sometimes this is for a reason. But often this kind of giving is done for no reason – 'just because'. There's a sense of excitement behind it where you just can't wait to tell that person or group what you've done for them or what you have for them. Even where your giving is anonymous, there's a feeling of rightness. This kind of giving feels light, playful and totally expansive.

The act of both types of giving, in theory, is the same, but the energy is completely different. If there were some magic device that could read and measure energy, wholeheartedness here would be 'off the Richter'.

Some people seem to be natural givers. They enjoy giving with their whole heart and expect absolutely nothing in return. Part of the reason might be chemistry – as we discovered in the previous chapter, in the section on the chemistry of connection, every time we give, we release a shot of oxytocin (a feel-good bonding hormone) into our system. And not only do you get a shot but the person you're giving to gets a shot, too. But it's not a conscious, clinical decision by us to release this feel-good hormone. It's deeper than that. The feel-good effects are just a by-product. We're designed to be givers. Because it feels good, yes, but also because it connects us.

We're not all natural givers – but we can all feel the joy of giving. We just need to start. The more we give, with our hearts in the right place, the more we cultivate an inner environment that yearns to give. The feeling is so fulfilling, we only want more of it. It's slightly addictive. In the best kind of way.

205

A few Christmases ago, I was on the way back to Sydney with my little cousin, Jessie, in the car. We'd had a lovely family Christmas in the country – with the few usual family dramas of course – and were driving along the Hume Highway just outside of Gundagai towards Sydney when I pulled into the famous 'Dog on the Tuckerbox' stop for fuel and a few cheeky refreshments. (What's a road trip without a bag of lollies?)

It was busy, only a few days after Christmas, and there were more people fuelling up and refreshing than normal. After filling the tank, I waited in line, Jessie by my side, until we finally arrived at the register and the woman behind the counter said, 'All good. Someone's paid for your fuel today.'

I'm not proud to admit this but the first thought that came into my mind was, 'Where's the creep and what does he want?' I just assumed that this 'guy' (although for all I knew, it could just as easily have been an elderly woman!) was just doing the old hit-on-the-blondes thing disguised as chivalry (don't tell me you haven't had the same thought before!).

Jessie and I stared at each other in amazement and when it finally became clear that no one was expecting applause, or to be made a hero, let alone get a phone number, I instantly felt alive with goodness. From the inside out.

A few other people near us heard the conversation and were just as chuffed, the attendant was beaming with excitement to tell me the news and Jessie's eyes were even bigger and more lit up that they normally are.

We paid for our travel treats, walked slowly to our car – still in a little disbelief – and proceeded to talk about how lovely the experience was for at least an hour.

In an instant, that anonymous giver created magic for everyone in that petrol station. I only hope the giver 'got' just as much as he or she gave. I hope they were just as high.

The story doesn't finish there.

Jessie and I made a commitment to pay it forward and both do a random act of kindness for a stranger in the coming weeks – anonymously.

It felt oh-so-good.

And it continues to feel good. 'RAK' is now a staple at the top of my weekly to-do list. I've left a single flower on someone's desk at the library; paid for many a coffee-lover's morning ritual in random places I only visit once (these are best done on holidays or road trips); left a copy of my favourite book on the train with a note inside greeting a stranger and telling them to 'enjoy'; and whatever else comes to me that time and that week. There are some weeks where a RAK doesn't eventuate and if it starts to feel like a chore I give it a break because I want it to always come from the heart. It's one of the most worthwhile things I can do with my time.

And I think giving anonymously is a great experiment in creating that steady and stunning flow of give and take. Just watch what happens when you give and expect nothing in return. Giving and being of service in the simplest and smallest of ways – whether anonymous or not – is profound.

own
the
flow

RANDOM ACTS OF KINDNESS

Set a few goals and a reminder to 'give' consciously through random acts of kindness over three consecutive weeks and see what happens. You could give anonymously, or the giving could be in your gestures. Give to people you know well, colleagues or family members, or to complete strangers. It's simple. And profound.

Some ideas to get you started:

A handwritten note for someone telling them you hope they have a great day and that something truly awesome happens for them.

A single flower on someone's windscreen.

Pay for a coffee for a stranger. Go to the barista, hand them the amount for a latte and say, 'The next person that comes in and orders one, tell them it's taken care of.' Smile and leave. (Or look for a café with a 'Pay It Forward' board that records pre-paid coffees for people who can't afford to buy their own.)

Let someone else in line before you.

Make something for someone.

Thank someone from your past or present for making a difference to your life (perhaps it's an old school teacher, a friend who was always kind to you, or your mother for caring for you all those years).

Help out at a homeless shelter but tell none of your friends or family members that you're doing it. It's not about you.

Donate to a charity – even a small amount makes a difference.

As you pass someone, send them a tiny silent blessing like, 'I wish you peace and joy today.' Go with whatever comes up and trust that it will hit them just the right way.

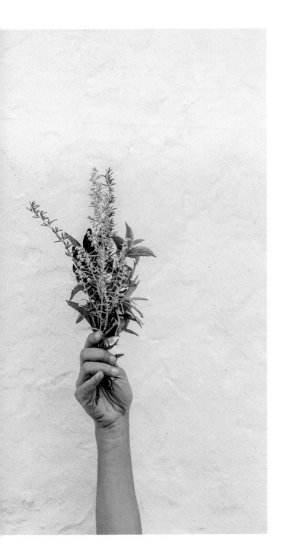

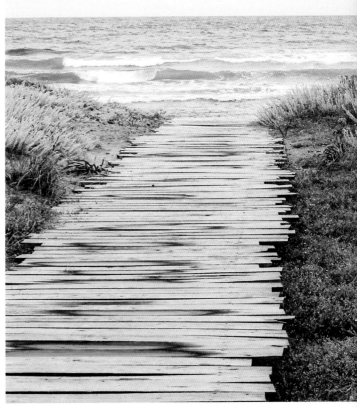

How to give wholeheartedly
– even if we're not feeling it

So what about the times when giving doesn't feel 'wholehearted' or authentic? After all, if the intention behind the giving is so important, why give when there's no good to give?

Because...

Sometimes we've just gotta. Because it's the 'right' thing to do. Because you'll save yourself the belly ache of not doing so. Or because sometimes – and I don't know what your circumstance or how this is hitting you right now – it can soften a relationship or be the beginnings of a humble reunion.

Here are some suggestions.

Let's say someone is rubbing you up the wrong way and you don't feel like giving your time and energy (cash doesn't even need to come into it). How about starting with a silent blessing?

 'Thank you for the lesson you're bringing to my life. This situation in which I feel stuck and blocked is being held up in front of me as a mirror reflecting exactly what it is that I still need to work on.'

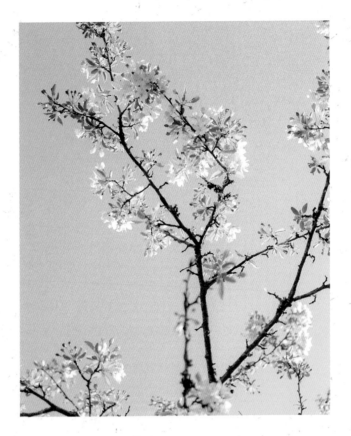

It doesn't mean that you're right and they are wrong or that you're the better person for giving. It's actually an exercise in surrender. You're loosening your grip on the angst you have in relation to that person. Soften on the situation and watch it change. It's not giving in. It's giving the situation over to some great mysterious force that has greater organising power than you could ever know. Work with it. Not against it.

Or perhaps there's a gift that you have to buy for another, but it feels like an obligation. How about investing in a charity for them? That way you get to choose a cause that you believe in and want to put positive energy behind, while also bypassing inauthenticity.

Giving to self – self care and all that jazz

What comes first? The chicken or the egg?

You know that saying that we have to apply our own oxygen mask before we can help others? I think that's true. But sometimes, it helps me to get the flow, energy, prana or chi moving when I'm in a downward place or spiral by giving to someone else. Then I feel good and can turn the energy around to give to myself.

And after all, when giving to others, we're giving to self, right?

So my conclusion is that, again, there needs to be an even flow of give and take, but if there isn't an intrinsic, deep-down love and appreciation of self, the giving can come across as inauthentic or it can deplete us.

Self care is something that hasn't come naturally to me since those earlier teenage years with anorexia. But it's not my fault. It's no one's.

I think we're born with a natural inclination to care. We're here for connection and a huge part of that connection is made up of caring for self and one another. But somewhere along the way, the care can become confused. What was once clear becomes clouded with competition.

Let's start with what self-care really is.

If a hot bath with Epsom salts after a decadent massage comes to mind – I reckon you're only part way there. Self-care goes way beyond pampering, eating nourishing food and taking your vitamins.

Self-care is…

Forgiving yourself when you screw up.

Loving yourself when you've had your heart broken.

Self-soothing on those long dark nights.

Feeling your way through tricky emotions without numbing yourself with alcohol, drugs, food or sex.

Choosing mentally uplifting and conscious conversation over gossip.

Self-care cultivates the following qualities….

Expansiveness

Love – the deep, deep kind (for self and others)

Integrity

Confidence

Clarity

Expressiveness

'Groundedness' or stability

Certainty

Self-care refuels rather than drains us.

And this is where that oxygen mask analogy can come in handy. For those of us who 'care' for others for a living, there can be a tendency to over-care, to the detriment of our own health.

I'm talking nurses, doctors, yoga teachers, charity workers, parents or guardians (females are particularly susceptible), community workers and so on. When we give more to others in this role, without giving back consciously to self, we begin to frazzle, wilt and burn out, big time.

Giving can become an addiction, a form of busy and another numbing mechanism for dealing with what's going on. We can tend to bury ourselves in our dharma or life's work as a way of running from our own 'stuff'.

My good mate and business partner, Benny, lost his mum to cancer. Around the anniversary of her death there's always an extra tenderness to him. He reflects, honours and remembers her, without fail and once, when I was going through my own burn-out, told me he thinks the reason the 'dis'-ease got the better of her in the end was because there was an imbalance in the give-take. She spent too much time giving. But never to herself. She had six kids to look after and was a nurse, always nurturing others. I've always remembered that and thought that, if I want to be able to keep 'giving' through my dharma of teaching yoga, I need to be able to self-care. Regularly.

For sustainability in our chosen form of service, we must give to self. It means getting better at saying 'no' with conviction and clarity and it means constantly re-assessing what it is to be balanced, physically and energetically.

Self-care can start with designated and disciplined rituals such as yoga practice, hot baths, morning meditations and nourishing meals. The effects then seep out into other aspects of life such as integrity in words (taking care that they aren't harming those around you);

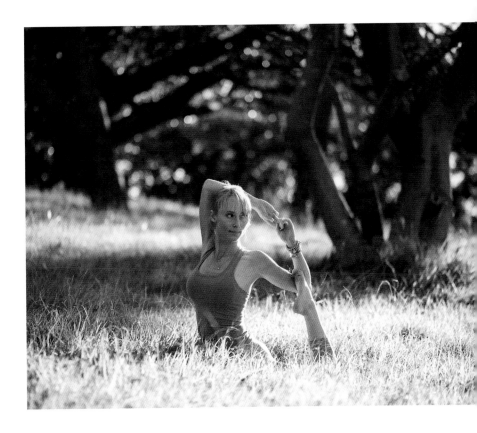

self-soothing when you know you've been triggered; and choosing to love yourself even in the middle of a break up, or other situations that might make you doubt your worth. These are all choices: choices to care and stay 'at home' in the body, rather than choosing escape and avoidance.

Self-care is the springboard for self-respect.

Self-care is the act of grounding and getting clear in the body – knowing your worth. And it allows you to walk the walk and not just talk the talk.

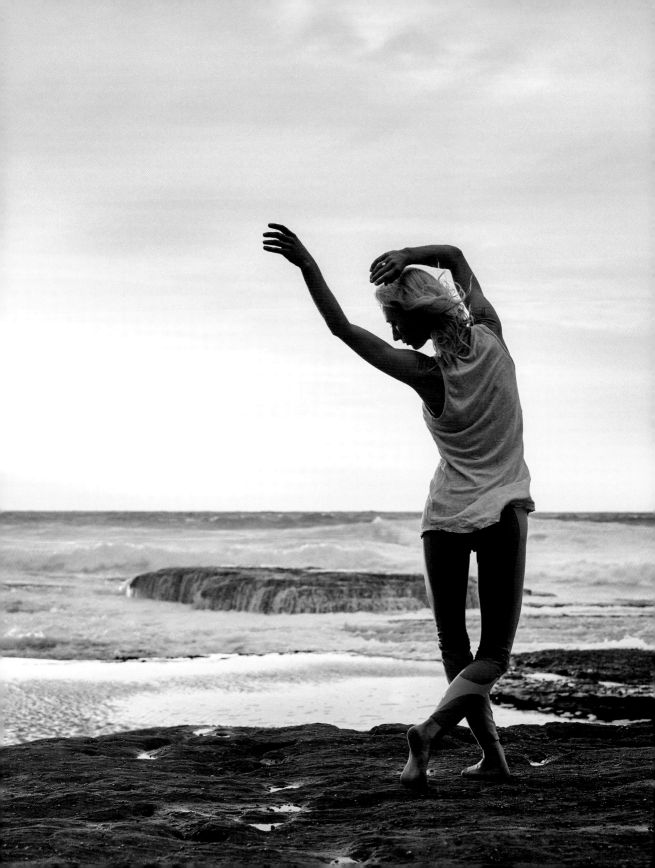

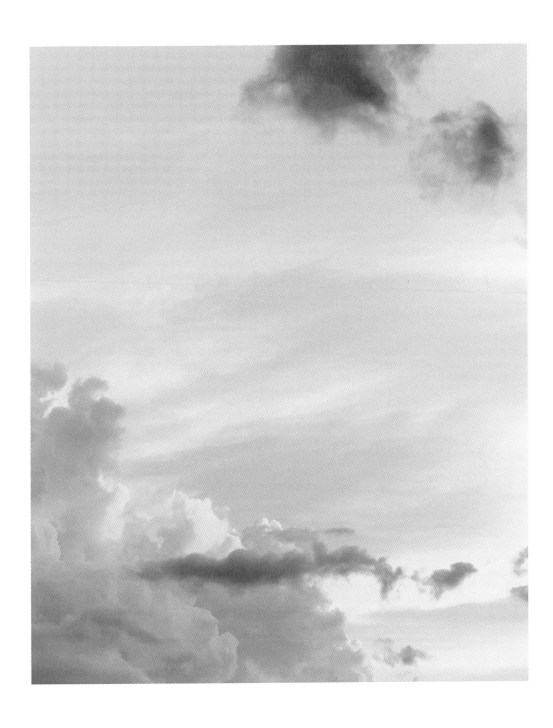

PHILOSOPHY 101.

The Intersect:

Where the Yin meets the Yang and the Yang meets the Yin

According to the Tantric Yoga view (which by the way is wayyyyy more than just sexual energy), energy flows between the two opposites, masculine and feminine, just as electric current flows between a negative and positive pole. The higher the voltage, the stronger the intensity of the current.

The same applies to sexual energy: in order for it to flow, we need two opposite poles – and the higher the difference, the stronger the energy is.

Different names have been used to describe the sexual poles:

Yin/Yang

Negative/Positive

Lunar/Solar

Shiva/Shakti

Whether you're male or female, you have both of these energies. To balance them out, or rather, to know when to lean into one aspect over the other, is the most fluid and beautiful dance you can be a part of.

It's about the masculine honouring the feminine and the feminine honouring the masculine.

Masculine energy doesn't have anything to do with being a man. Nor is feminine energy only found in women. Here are some rough distinctions that show the polar opposites of both:

Masculine Energy v Feminine Energy

Doing v Being

Active v Surrender

Analytical v Intuitive

Left Brain v Right Brain

Assertive v Receptive

Striving v Becoming

Logical v Creative

Hard v Soft

Controlling v Allowing

Women can tap into their masculine energy to get things done and men can tap into the feminine to fulfil creative roles or make decisions on the felt sense of intuition.

We've become so fast and 'results-driven' in today's society and are so often rewarded for 'getting the job done' that we tend to lean into our masculine more than we need to. I'm talking to you if you've ever experienced burn-out – no matter how mild or crushing. The masculine keeps us in a constant state of action, which – over time – is depleting.

On the other end of the spectrum if we lean into the feminine for too long we can get a bit 'head in the clouds', or become goal-less. We can feel unproductive and unfulfilled, which is also one of the most crushing feelings for a human being.

Knowing when to lean into each of the polarities is a skill that takes practice. And I'm still practising, each day. I assume I will be all my life.

It's the delicate dance between the masculine and feminine, the 'doing' with the 'being', that makes it all so interesting.

Another way to illustrate these two polar energies is to look at the Yin Yang symbol.

 Yang is white, male, hot, directional, active, dynamic, solid, dense.

Yin is black, female, cool, resting, vast, timeless, eternal, liquid.

In life, as in love, the qualities of Yin and Yang are in a constant interplay, weaving in and out of each other as a continual evolutionary dance. When you understand this, you no longer have to manifest a war of the sexes. You can allow the weaving of Yin and Yang elements to move and play and enjoy learning from each other through this interchange.

In the Yin Yang symbol, the black area represents Yin, the white area Yang. However, within the white is a black dot. And within the black is a white dot. This illustrates that if you go totally into Yin it will lead you to Yang. And if you go totally into Yang, it will lead you to Yin.

If I use the idea of Yin and Yang to look at our current situation and what's been happening here and around the world, I see that for so long there's been a super-strong masculine energy of 'doing' and destroying. We see it in politics, what we're doing to the environment and how we treat each other – after all, how we do one thing is how we do all, right? There's been an imbalance between the sexes, but all of that is starting to shift. I really do believe that more people on the planet are starting to lead from their feminine side, using their heart.

I am not saying that men are to blame for women having felt the underdog in many spheres for so long. In fact, women have a huge role to play in politics, law and other traditionally male-dominated industries, but perhaps the problem has been that women in these roles have felt that they've needed to lean too far into their masculine to make a difference.

And this is where, I think, we've gone wrong.

It's the feminine that's needed in these roles to make top-of-culture decisions based on the good of all. In other words, males and females could lean into creative and intuitive thinking to make worldly decisions, rather than black and white, masculine 'I'm right, you're wrong' kinds of decisions.

And in love, an area where I've had many a life lesson, this is what I've learnt:

When a woman allows a man to be a man – without wanting to change, nag or push him into a sensitivity he's not ready for – she allows him to be his brightest self. And when a man allows a woman to be a woman, in all of her sensitivity and softness, she feels her most divine self. And when the balance is there; when the dance is being danced (consciously), the relationship falls into an effortless state of ease. The man feels like a man. The woman feels like the woman. The man is no longer afraid to dip into his vulnerabilities because something has unlocked. The woman isn't afraid to stand up for herself and create boundaries. Because something has been unlocked.

It's in the allowing. The 'I'll do me and you do you'.

When I'm full and inhabiting the whole of my body, unashamedly, I give permission for you to do the same.

And that cultivates honour, respect and a deep, deep kind of love. It's where two really become one.

It's all part of this great mystery.

Intention and manifestation

Intention setting is a huge part of my self-practice, and something I encourage my students to do.

With an intention, we channel energy like a river in the direction of our dreams.

Where we reap the benefits of this intention depends on where we direct the intention.

At the beginning of my asana practice, I'll set an intention that is either self-based or dedicated to something or someone else – but as we know, there is no separation between the individual and other so it's all same, same.

When applying it to practice, intention can be broken down into two types – neither superior to the other because whether they seem to be expressed outwardly or inwardly, they both involve cultivating a flow of giving and receiving.

In a **self-based** intention, I generally get clear on a bhavna or feeling state that I wish to evoke, often related to my values as a yogi. For example, I may wish to set an intention to feel 'light'. The idea, then, is that I take this word and bring it into my practice in such a way that I embody it. I like to imagine that if anyone were watching me, they'd be able to see that I'm practising 'lightness'. Light in the way I move, breathe and sense things. Light in the way I react to falling out of a posture or not quite nailing something I could do well last week.

I embody it.

And because there is no clear line that marks where my practice begins and finishes, from mat to 'real world', I take this intention with me. Then all my decisions – who I spend time with that day, the words I speak, the actions I take – are all in line with this intention to cultivate 'light'. The giving in this experiment is that I share 'light' with those around me. The light becomes my act of service and how I give to the world and those around me that day.

My intention is my devotion.

When practising this kind of intention and being disciplined enough to stay aligned to it, we see just how creative we are as human beings. We can imagine something, a state in this case, and we can either have it in our hands or feel completely surrounded by it. We've manifested it. And that's pure magic.

The **self-less** kind of intention, if set before asana practice, could be that I'm dedicating the next hour on the mat to someone who really needs it. Perhaps I have a friend who's going through a hard time and needs some extra support. I'll dedicate practice to that person and perhaps infuse it with a bhavna or feeling state like 'love' or 'comfort' or 'joy', whatever I feel, intuitively, that they need.

You don't need the four corners of a yoga mat for setting intention, however.

You can wake up each day and decide how you're going to feel and what or who you're going to be of service to that day. All it requires is a quiet moment to ground, an awareness of your connection to all things and your quiet words of dedication.

And your dedication doesn't always have to go deep – especially when it feels forced, or a strain.

If today, you just intend to endeavour to be calmer and more grounded, then so be it. Simplicity is often key.

If you practise Ashtanga and your intention is to, over a period of time, advance from 'Ashtanga Primary' to 'Ashtanga Intermediate', it will happen one way or the other.

If your intention is to become stronger, master the most difficult asanas, hold your breath for more than a minute, and release toxins through the practice, it will definitely provide you with these benefits, too.

Aim for what you need on that day – just always remember that the practice of yoga is much more than the physical. So set the physical goals, if that's what's calling you. But perhaps also get clear on the desired feeling as an outcome. Not only will this kind of intention bring you more fulfilment, daily, but you may have a chance of reaching that physical manifestation more quickly.

Why?

Because if we're conscious of attracting that intended feeling and staying close to the reason why we want to feel that way, it's a practice in magnetisation. Cultivating that feeling state, day by day, brings you far closer to the manifestation.

A practice without intention is empty. A practice with intention towards a physical or material goal is limited to only that.

A practice with intention towards a spiritual goal is unlimited in its possibilities.

Yoga is a path to freedom or moksha (a term in Hinduism, Buddhism and Jainism that means liberation or release). It's a path to balance our emotions, health and mind. It helps us to feel good about ourselves and ultimately transforms the body. But above all, yoga means union – a merging with the divine. It is a spiritual practice to transform all aspects of our lives in order to merge with something greater than our limited sense of self.

The process – from intention to manifestation

It's one thing to set an intention and then expect that, boom, it's right there in front of you or that you're going to achieve an acquired bhavna or feeling state all day. I wish. How easy would that be?

As I say to my students after a class in which we have set intentions, 'take the practice with you'.

And by that I mean…

Take your intention and live by it; act by it; speak by it; embody it.

After all, how we do one thing is how we do all.

The divine is in the detail.

If my intention on a particular day is to 'care deeply', I'm going to care deeply about doing the dishes. I'm going to care deeply about conversing with a friend, stranger or loved one. I'm going to care deeply about my food choices. I'm going to care deeply about where that pair of jeans that I have my eye on really comes from. Did the manufacturers care deeply about their staff?

Sounds like a lot of work, ha? At first, perhaps. But then attention to detail and deep care become a natural part of your daily selection. Everything you do gets wrapped up in integrity.

There's a magic formula to intention setting and having it manifest in various ways. And it goes like this:

One.

Set the intention.

Two.

Let go of how it comes to be. You don't have to know every step of the way. Lean into the mystery and...

Three.

Follow the charm. Allow yourself to be pulled by the things that give resonance to your intention. And once truly charmed or pulled towards something, trust and...

Four.

Take action. Stay aligned to the value and live it in each moment. This takes effort, but the discipline always creates freedom. Even if it doesn't feel like it in the moment.

'Those whose consciousness is unified abandon all attachment to the results of action and attain supreme peace. But those whose desires are fragmented, who are selfishly attached to the results of their work, are bound in everything they do,' says *The Bhagavad Gita*, an ancient Hindu scripture

And if things don't quite work out the way you hoped, remember that one day you may stand back and marvel at the grand plan that 'the great mystery' had in store for you instead. Somehow, it always knows the way and has a plan far more imaginative than you or I could muster up for ourselves. I absolutely know this to be true.

Magic is everywhere, if only we'd open our eyes to it.

mantra | being of service

When practising this sequence, have an intention in mind. What is it that you wish to dedicate your practice to? Is there someone or some great cause that could do with the focus and care that you generate through these gentle and mindful movements?

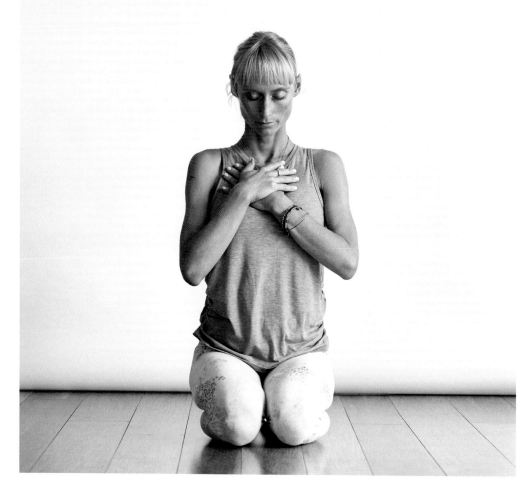

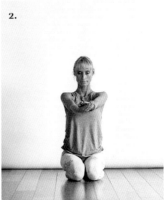

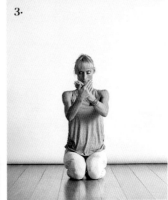

Take the first round super slow with around five breaths per posture and then for each round after that it's one breath per movement, so that it really begins to flow and take on the feeling of a slow, fluidly flowing moving meditation.

1 Virasana (hands on heart) From a kneeling posture (placing a block or cushion under the sit bones if you feel uncomfortable in the hips, ankles or feet), press down into the tops of the feet to the ground. Lengthen the spine gently and place one hand on top of the other over the heart. Take five deep breaths with eyes closed.

2 Arms Extend Inhale, and extend the arms out in front, keeping that one hand on top of the other. On full extension the palm of the bottom hand faces up.

3 Hands Back to Heart Exhale. Bring the hands (one on top of other) back to the heart.

4a.

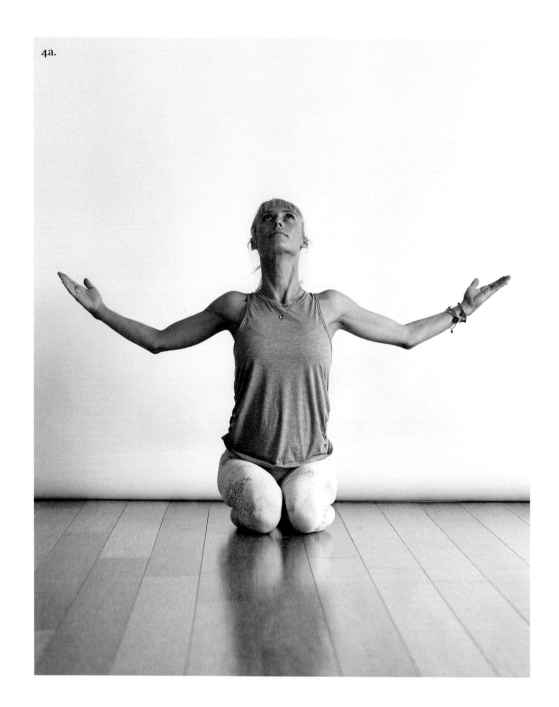

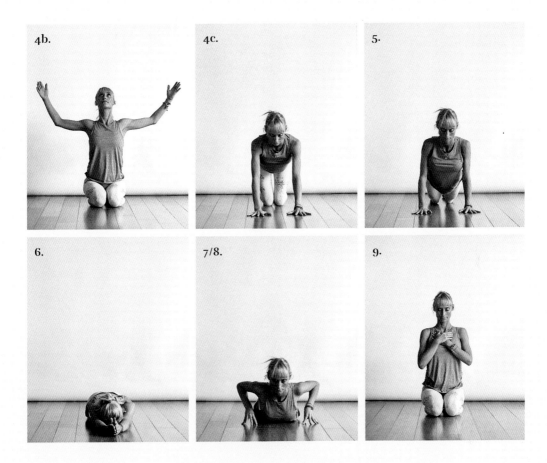

4b.   4c.   5.

6.   7/8.   9.

4 Inhale, taking the hands out in front so that you're on all fours.

5 Exhale down to the ground so that the chest lands and then the abdomen.

6 Inhale, lengthening the arms out into full prostration.

7 Exhale. Slide the hands back underneath the shoulders.

8 Inhale. Ease the chest forwards and up into a baby cobra as you internally rotate the thighs and gently point back into the toes.

9 Exhale back into kneeling, returning the hands, one hand on top of the other, over the heart.

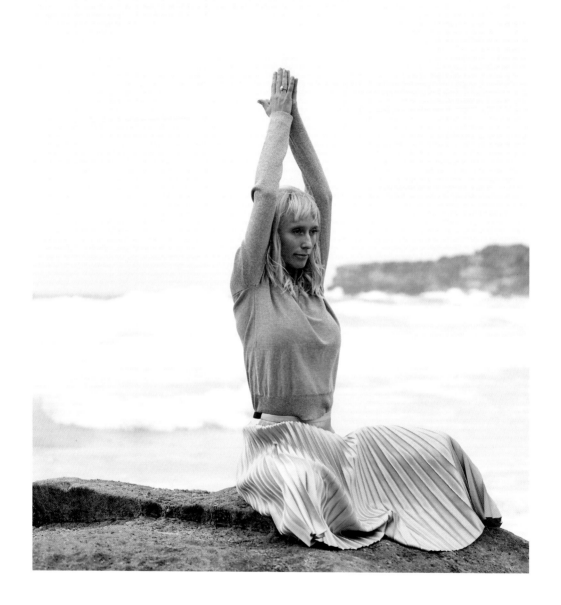

Dharma

Your calling as your life's work

'Your work is to discover your work and then with all your heart to give yourself to it.' Buddha

As I said previously, diversification in devotion is required to have a global community that cares. Not only for one another but for every corner of the planet.

Sometimes I imagine each of us to be uniquely imprinted with a worthy cause that will serve the world and that figuring out that cause, and living it out, will be one of our greatest accomplishments in life.

My very first yoga class was at the Dharma Shala in North Bondi. And when, in my increasingly obsessed stages of my early yoga years, I looked up the meaning of the name, I learnt a lot.

Dharma is a word found in both Buddhism and Hinduism.

To a Buddhist, dharma is the essential teachings to transform the mind towards that of an enlightened being. And as such...

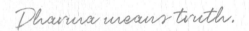
Dharma means truth.

It's not just rituals such as lighting candles, reading scriptures or visiting a temple. It's what we take with us out into the every day. Dharma is the way of living that we devote our lives to; specifically, in the Buddhist tradition, this comes down to living with compassion and kindness. It's about living the truth. Living your truth.

Remember, the divine is in the details.

In Hinduism (and explored in the Vedas – made up of four classical Hinduism texts) it's implied that only the sages could experience dharma and it was their 'service' or work to pass on their knowledge to others through mantras and actions. Later, however, the writings known as Dharma Sutras gave a different meaning and indicated that dharma was the performance of duties in accordance to the Vedic law. Dharma was taking on one's role in Vedic society.

The latter makes way more sense and offers tonnes of hope and fulfilment for us mere mortals.

And the Sanskrit word shala means house or home.

How fitting that the Dharma Shala was not only the first place I took an asana class, but also proved to be the beginning of an epic journey of self-discovery. It would lead me to a life of yoga as being my most fulfilling act of service to the world. To date, at least – because the way we carry out our truths, with integrity, passion and clarity, can change. In 10 years' time, I may be doing something quite different. But I have a hunch the 'feeling' will remain the same.

I didn't always have this kind of clarity around what I wanted to do. I went straight from school to university – I even knocked back a trip offered to me so generously by my mum to go to Italy for a gap year. I decided to go straight on to more studying because all my friends were doing that. Was I crazy?

I studied Media and Cultural Studies at Macquarie University because it was the thing that lit me up most at the time. What I would do with it though – I had no clue. But I followed the charm.

Straight out of university I got lucky and scored a great job with a wicked team of guys I'm blessed enough to call family. It was fun, but I knew it wasn't my life's purpose, or dharma. However, during this time I did start to practise yoga – a lot. And my job in that little creative agency funded that new addiction.

So if you don't think you're living your dharma – don't stress. I reckon you're on the path in one way or another. You've just got to trust. And keep following the charm.

If you look back from where you're at right now you might see that although some things didn't seem, at the time, as though they turned out your way, in hindsight, they happened so perfectly.

This has definitely been true in my own experience of the finding of my life's purpose. Here's what I've learnt.

Finding your dharma has a lot to do with 'feeling'. And by that I mean…

We're all striving for goals and so-called success. But at the very core of all of that is a desired feeling. We want to get that promotion at work because we want to feel 'alive'; we want to buy that house so that we'll feel 'stable'; we want to be in a healthy relationship because we want to feel 'loved'.

When we dig even deeper into these feelings, there's an undertone of freedom, or moksha, and that feels expansive. There's expansion in feeling alive, loved and stable. There's expansiveness in feeling recognised, sexy or confident. And as long as we're not attached to these feelings for our self-worth, expansiveness is the gift that keeps on giving. It motivates us to give to others and to feel trusting of the world around us.

So I'd argue – extensively – that although we may have different words for it, we're all working towards the freedom we feel in expansiveness. And when we find that in our life's work, we go next level. When we're acting from a place of expansiveness, unrestrained by obligation, we fall into the flow of life. And that's the whole point.

So what makes you feel expansive?

Identify it. And follow it. It might take you many years to find your calling, but with enough belief and a wide-awake mind and heart, you will find it.

And P.S. Your dharma doesn't have to be that thing that you do that earns you a living. It could be that you're an accountant by day and you make scarves for the poor at night. Because that makes you feel expansive.

Or maybe you are an accountant and that feels expansive.

I once heard Eckhart Tolle, a spiritual teacher and writer, talk in Sydney and I remember him saying that 'expansiveness is our natural state'. I believe that to be true.

It was this feeling of expansiveness that led me to my own dharma.

To illustrate, let me recall three very clear and 'expansive' moments. Moments in which time stood still and I could almost feel my cells expand, merge and dissolve into the atmosphere around me.

 First.

I was in high school. Circa year eight. I was one of those kids that was friends with everyone – the boarders, the day girls, the girls in the years above and below, and somehow the teachers found me funny and liked me, too. I was lucky (and a little cheeky) but I was also a dedicated student and worked hard. I didn't naturally get good grades like some of my friends. I had to work at it.

My school was a big, old convent. I remember the room we were in at this particular moment. Sandstone walls, filled with girls all starting to stress about some upcoming exams. We were given 10 minutes at the end of class to discuss a pending exam and fire questions at our teacher, Mr McDonough. He was getting clearly frustrated with the nature of some of the questions and the girls increasingly worked up. I saw an opportunity to make a joke – I don't even remember what it was – so I did. Must have been semi-funny, because all of a sudden the whole room was lit up with laughter – including Mr McDonough's.

It was the first of those expansive moments, even though I wasn't aware enough to label it that way back then. For just a few moments, everyone in the room was in hysterics. My fellow students had all dropped their concerns and the teacher's frustration had vanished. For one moment, everyone in the room was in some way free from the past and future.

Everyone was present.

And for some reason that feeling really stayed with me.

 Second.

About 10 years later. I'm finishing up a morning class at the Dharma Shala, quickly changing and then heading out the door to jump on the bus into the city for work. Rick, my very first yoga teacher, hails me and says something that stops in my tracks. It will change the course of my life.

'You know, Katie, you'd make a really good yoga teacher, you should think about doing your teacher training.'

Every cell wide open. Alert and listening. Another expansive moment.

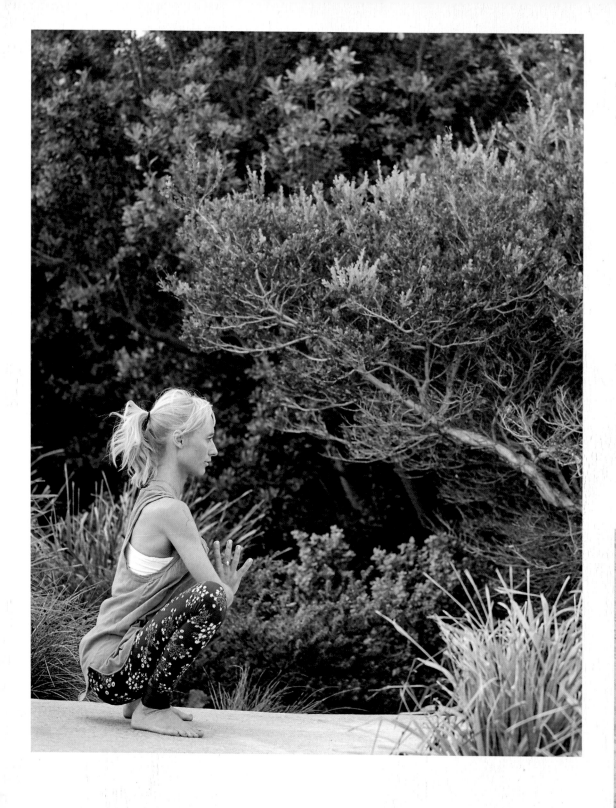

Third.

I'm teaching my first class at the Dharma Shala.

After doing my yoga teacher training in Goa, India, I'd come back doubtful that I could make a living from teaching and flirted for a few months with the idea of working full-time back in the advertising industry. Thankfully I plucked up the courage to take a job teaching and worked up hours at gyms, smaller yoga studios and doing private lessons at people's houses. After about a year and a half Rick and I decided it was time to teach at the Shala.

I was nervous. Very. Many of the students I'd be teaching had been practising there for way longer than I had. What did I have to offer? What could I teach them?

But all those insecurities vanished after our opening chant. I started to expand. There was a moment half-way through class when I was facing the south side of the room thinking, this is it. I've arrived. I've expanded into and accepted my dharma. The hairs on my arms stood up.

And I still have this feeling of expansiveness when I'm teaching. It doesn't come without fear and insecurity at times. But the feeling I get when I teach far outweighs the fear.

There were points early on when I was freelancing, before Flow Athletic had opened, where I was exhausted from all the running around from one person's house to the other, from studio classes to working with athletes. For that time, there were most definitely days when that sense of expansiveness was lulled. It paid to listen to that feeling, too.

Listening to the feelings of contraction is just as relevant to finding almost anything you want, not just your dharma.

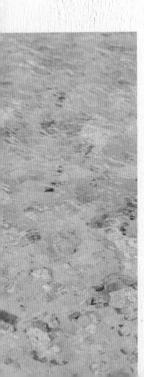

My feelings of lethargy, exhaustion and not wanting to get out of bed some mornings when I knew I had a big day were giving me important signals to change direction. It didn't mean to change jobs but rather just to change the nature of what I was doing.

I learnt from these moments that if I wanted to continue to be a yoga teacher as well as have all the experiences I desired in life, I was going to have to think outside the box. There was only one of me.

So the choice was either to work with other people to build a team that shared the same values and mission or (in my case 'and') be a little more entrepreneurial and adapt my skills outside of yoga to what I was doing.

I started writing more. I'd hassle the editors of health and wellness publications until they let me write for them and after much hustling landed a regular job with *Body + Soul* as their yoga content 'guru'. From there other doors opened and before I knew it, I was making a decent income outside of my yoga teaching and private classes.

When you know you were born to do something, you find a way.

Did I get push back along the way? Not so much with my teaching, but perhaps with Flow Athletic, yes. I remember one yoga teacher that I met in Bali putting her hand out to welcome me to the country she'd decided to live in. At the same time the person who was introducing us told her I owned a studio in Sydney and when our hands connected she looked me in the eyes and said, 'Oh, I'm sorry.' There's a belief in the yoga world that running a studio can be laborious and stifle that 'free spirit' mentality that comes with being a yogi. But if it's making you feel expansive, it's not limiting. It's freeing.

Creating opportunities for team members to also do what they love – that's expansive. Providing a space for students to come and practise yoga – a place where healing takes place and many 'aha' moments occur – that's expansive.

We're all diverse in our dharma.

What turns me on didn't turn this yoga teacher on. And that's the coolest part of all. We've all been karmically given a unique role to fulfil. And our states of expansiveness and contraction lead the way.

In fact, some of my most motivating of moments have come from times when people have told me I couldn't do something, or that what I was contemplating was not the right thing to do. I can be a sucker for listening to too many people, but on some rare occasions when very headstrong and successful people that I look up to and admire tell me 'no', the fire in my belly that comes from that word tells me it's a definite 'yes'. Everyone is in front of us for a reason.

Even the push back can set us free.

Whether it's knitting, child-minding, plumbing, running a global financial institution or opening your own meditation studio, you find a way to do what you love. You find a way to create expansion (or whatever other word you have for it).

Apple founder Steve Jobs once said that given our time is limited, we shouldn't waste it living someone else's lives – that we shouldn't let what he called 'the noise of other opinions' stop us following our hearts and our intuition. He was right.

Do what you love. Not what you think others want you to do or what's typically expected of you.

Lean in and listen to yourself.

Follow the charm.

Finding your dharma

So far, we've looked at the importance of being present and open to those states of expansion and contraction. In addition, there are a few ways that the yogi cultivates an environment that will encourage a life's purpose to show up and be crystal clear. They're through the 10 Laws of Dharma, set out in an ancient Hindu text.

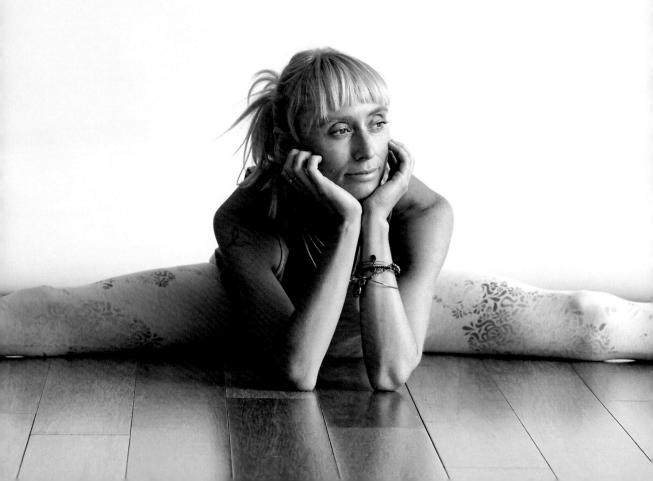

The 10 laws of dharma

The ancient sage Manu prescribed 10 essential observances of dharma.

Patience (dhriti) – Staying secure in your own inner peace.

Forgiveness (kshama) – Letting go of things that don't serve you.

Willpower (dama) – Knowing that the best things come to those who wait – we don't have to take every single opportunity. Go with what feels truly right instead.

Honesty (asteya) – Let this honesty come up in speech and actions. Walking the walk, not just talking the talk, gives you bargaining power way beyond what you can imagine.

Cleanliness (shaucha) – Purity in mind, body and soul. This also takes willpower and a sense of self-devotion.

Control of senses (indraiya-nigrah) – Meditation and life force or 'prana' control.

Reason (dhi) – Guiding your life with calm reason leads to success.

Knowledge or Learning (vidya) – Gaining skills that significantly add to your ability to offer value to the world around you. How can you be of service?

Truthfulness (satya) – Realising that truthfulness brings about the highest outcome for you and others.

Absence of anger (krodha) – It's said that anger poisons our ability to lead our lives in a positive way. It encourages a life led in fear. Instead I like to replace this law with Non-Violence (ahimsa), which means non-harm to others and leading out of love.

Legacy

What is it that *you* will leave behind?

I remember someone asking me once: 'What would you want people to say about you when you're gone? And if you could attend your funeral, how would you want to feel? How would your family and friends honour you? How would they remember you?'

I think it's one of the most profound and insanely motivating questions I've been asked.

Whether we like it or not, death is approaching. Right now, as you take a breath, it's the most amount of breaths you've ever taken in your whole entire life. Every step you take creates a new total for how many steps you've taken in your life. So how are you treading and what's the footprint you're leaving behind?

What do you stand for?

Back around the time of Dad's funeral, I remember having a session with Michael Trembath, the energy healer mentioned in previous parts of this book. When discussing death, he mentioned that all our issues, addictions and hang ups dissolve to leave only the purest parts of you. I like to believe this to be true. Although we don't forget about the darkest parts of another person at death, as these made that person who they were with all their edges and scars, we honour and lean into what they left behind and how they made people feel.

So here goes. This is what I hope for at my funeral.

——————

That my family remembers me for the child that I was and still am. Playful, shy, active, resilient; not afraid to get dirty and have adventures beyond the perimeter of my home.

That I inspired a small community of people in Sydney to practise presence and cultivate a state of calm – and worldwide, too, through my online practices, books, yoga teacher training, posts and articles.

That I created soul-expanding experiences to help people to feel uplifted and more connected to themselves.

That my messaging was relevant, relatable and inspiring.

That my closest friends felt deeply loved and cared for by me and that they always felt they could share their deepest of secrets or shameful acts. When we share the shame (which can be the birth place of violence, bullying, self-harm and illness), that shame dissolves. A listening ear is important in this world.

That I was honest; that I spoke my truth and was courageous enough to give people my honest opinion.

That I was able to live my dharma wholeheartedly. That through my acts of service – teaching, educating people about, living and breathing my yoga – I was authentic and able to make a difference in some way to the people around me.

That members of my family felt at peace with our relationship and could always count on me. Mostly though, I hope they felt loved by me.

I hope my partner (who I care for in a way that is indescribable except for the fact that when I think of him as I write these words my heart swells up) will always remember the depth of our relationship and that I was forever changed for knowing him. I hope he knows that he slowly changed some of my negative patterns and beliefs just by loving me. Thank you for always telling me how lovable, beautiful and sexy I am. Even if, some days, I couldn't bring myself to believe you. It still mattered.

That strangers I met felt inspired to be mindful and calm.

And whilst sitting back and watching all of this after my spirit has left my body, I hope to feel liberated; that I know I gave all that I had to give and just as equally received all the gifts people, and the universe, wanted to give.

I hope to leave this world expansive, dissolving into and truly understanding my connection to it all.

———

What's your legacy?

Have a think about what you would want people to say at your funeral.

How would you feel upon hearing the words that are said?

Death is an imminent, crazy and beautiful thing. It really is a sweet reminder to live in a way that is authentic to you, that brings meaning to your life and that, in some way, encourages you to 'give' and to be of service – because that really is the most fulfilling way to walk the Earth.

Honour

Legacy and honour go hand in hand. The pairing circles back to that core belief that life is all about giving and receiving and the artful balance between the two.

Just as we may wish to leave a legacy behind (as grand or subtle and simple as it may be), we can honour those who have left behind a legacy of their own. They can inspire us to keep on keeping on when things get tough and we feel out of alignment. We can lean into their legacy, hoping to return – in some way – to our own.

Often, I'll lean into the legacy of other yoga teachers who have achieved what I hope to achieve. I'll lean into the legacy of my partner who is remarkable in his approach to his passion.

The nature of the legacy that I lean into varies. Sometimes I thirst for tenderness, in which case I look to my friend Maryanne, and the gentle manner in which she approaches her teaching, relationships and nieces. Sometimes it's fire in the belly, in which case I honour another mate, Pammy.

Inspiration is everywhere.

Yogi 4

MY MUMMA

On Mother's Day this year, I honoured my mum and gave thanks for all the lessons I've learnt under her 'daughter-hood'.

Although I was honouring a parent, I was also honouring what it is to be a mother and the energy that's cultivated from it. So, while I was honouring Jan Kendall, I was also honouring the feminine aspect in each of us – men included.

As discussed earlier in the book, according to Tantric Yoga philosophy, we all have a feminine and masculine energy and although my mum can seem to take on the role of the masculine sometimes (she's fiery, active and was most certainly the disciplinarian out of the two of my parents), on this day, I decided to honour her feminine side. The side that really made me feel cared for and loved. Unconditionally.

This is part of what I wrote in a blog post dedicated to her.

To celebrate and honour my own mother (who, by the way, sacrificed so damn much), here are a few words:

Thank you for sharing and teaching your adventurous spirit, fun-loving attitude and the belief that you're never too old to be a kid.

I love you more than you can know and every time I think of you I count my lucky stars and thank you for all that you sacrificed so that I could have so many incredible opportunities. I like to think they paid off and that I've made you proud.

You taught me the importance of good work ethics and that 'a job worth doing is worth doing well'; that a bag of Liquorice Allsorts is a delight; and to hold my breath when the Sydney Swans are in a tight game.

Biggest of love, Mumma, your Kate.

I concluded the post with this:

May each day feel like Mother's Day. Be kind to yourself. If you don't, no one else will.

Conclusion

As I sit to wrap this book up in words and send you off inspired to truly 'let go', to catch the current of whatever waves decide to pick you up in this moment and live a life in flow, I've – only days ago – given birth to a beautiful little girl. She's all the inspiration I need to write this: a perfect reminder that life is precious. Blink and we miss it. Right now, I stare into her barely open eyes and realise that before I know it she'll have children of her own.

It is never too late to start living the life you want.

We can press the reset button each morning to reinvent ourselves. Daily.

Remember that rituals are a deep reverence to self and a way to slow down and to savour life's moments. How fully can you pour yourself into the ones that make you feel like you are you but, more importantly, remind you of your connection to all beings and things?

Yoga is sacred movement but also a playful way to stay in tune to your body's needs and the environment around it. Take your body out into nature – often. May it be far more interested in what trees it shall climb today than the outfit it will wear to work.

Remember what brings you joy and lean into those things, never underestimating the power of a good belly laugh. But don't forget to honour sadness and grief, too, as another way to feel more connected to this human experience.

And speaking of connection, remember that we're all made up of the same stuff and we're all going through our own highs and lows. Make like a Buddhist and practise kindness and compassion. When someone cuts you off in traffic or jumps in front in the coffee queue, remember what's really important. Maybe they have a lot on their mind or they just didn't notice you. Mistakes happen.

Whenever possible (and it's always possible), let's make our relationships deeper and more meaningful. Listen - with every cell. Because sometimes the greatest gift you can give is to let someone be heard.

If I look across to my daughter right now, I wish for her a life in which she experiences an abundance of love and playfulness and is open to the experiences that this great mystery has to offer her.

This mystery has grander plans that I can even imagine for her or that she might dream up for herself one day. Surrender is the key. This surrender is the same wish I have for myself and for all of us.

We can plan and hustle all we like but, in the end, I think we're all just being 'done'. Allow it to happen and experience pure magic.

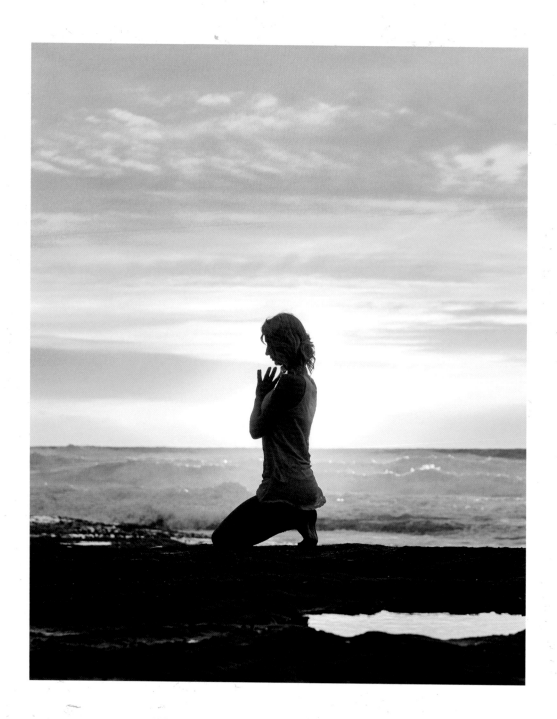

Thanks

To my very first yoga teacher, Rick Barnsdale. Thank you for inspiring my practice and for encouraging me in those early days. You and the Dharma Shala will always hold a very special place in my heart.

Ben Lucas – for believing in me when I didn't and for encouraging me to do big things – like write a book.

Amanda Prior, Bianca Cheah and Chen Ryan – thank you for catching my best angles and for the many photographs you contributed to this book. And to the whole Murdoch Books team. You made the experience so fun and smooth. I absolutely loved working with you, especially Kelly Doust, who took a chance.

Andrew Johns – you're more of a yogi than you know. Many of the pages in this book on joy, connection and love are an ode to you. It all started with a few yoga classes and now we have a beautiful baby girl. I couldn't love you both any more. But I will.

Ella and Kirrily – thanks for tirelessly helping me spread my message. You've helped me do big things.

Macca – thanks for all the belly laughs. Some of the best medicine I ever had.

Michael Trembath and Megan Trembath – for keeping me balanced.

Chris, Damian and the whole team from Aro Hā Wellness Adventure Retreat, for reminding me to reset and immerse myself in nature often. The space you hold on that mountain is nothing short of magic.

And finally, to anyone who has taken a yoga class of mine before, as well as my regular legends on the mat at Flow Athletic. Thank you for trusting me to hold space and for letting me do what I love most.

Sources

Chapter 1

1 Jerath, R., Edry J.W, Barnes, V.A. & Jerath, V. (2006). Physiology of long pranayamic breathing: Neural respiratory elements may provide a mechanism that explains how slow deep breathing shifts the autonomic nervous system. *Medical Hypothesis*, 67, 566-571.

Chapter 2

1 Emmons, R. A. & McCullough, M. E. (2003). Counting blessings versus burdens: Experimental studies of gratitude and subjective well-being in daily life. *Journal of Personality and Social Psychology*, 84, 377-389.

2 Emmons, R. A. & Mishra, A. (2012). Why gratitude enhances well-being: What we know, what we need to know. In Sheldon, K., Kashdan, T., & Steger, M.F. (eds.) *Designing the future of positive psychology: Taking stock and moving forward*. New York: Oxford University Press.

Chapter 3

1 Stiner, M.C. & Kuhn, S.L. (2009). Paleolithic Diet and the Division of Labor in Mediterranean Eurasia. In: Hublin J.J. & Richards M.P. (eds) *The Evolution of Hominin Diets. Vertebrate Paleobiology and Paleoanthropology*. Springer, Dordrecht. www.researchgate.net/publication/225948255_Paleolithic_Diet_and_the_Division_of_Labor_in_Mediterranean_Eurasia

2 Oarizh, D. (2002). Speed of Nerve Impulses. hypertextbook.com/facts/2002/DavidParizh.shtml

3 Heart Foundation. How Your Heart Works. www.heartfoundation.org.au/your-heart

4 Walter, C. (2012). Affairs of the Lips. *Scientific American*. www.scientificamerican.com/article/affairs-of-the-lips-2012-10-23/

5 Kuehni, R.G. (2015). How many object colors can we distinguish? Wiley Online Library onlinelibrary.wiley.com/doi/full/10.1002/col.21980

6 Bergland, C. (2012). The Neurochemcials of Happiness, *Psychology Today*, www.psychologytoday.com/au/blog/the-athletes-way/201211/the-neurochemicals-happiness

7 Kuss, D.J. & Griffiths, M.D. (2011). Online Social Networking and Addiction — A Review of the Psychological Literature. *Int J Environ Res Public Health*. 2011 Sep; 8(9): 3528–3552. www.ncbi.nlm.nih.gov/pmc/articles/PMC3194102/

8 Kuss, D.J. & Griffiths, M.D. (2017). Social Networking Sites and Addiction: Ten Lessons Learned *Int J Environ Res Public Health* 2017 Mar 17;14(3). pii: E311. www.ncbi.nlm.nih.gov/pubmed/28304359

9 Raghunathan, R. (2013). How Negative is Your Mental Chatter? *Psychology Today*, www.psychologytoday.com/us/blog/sapient-nature/201310/how-negative-is-your-mental-chatter

10 Cascio, C.N., O'Donnell M.B., Tinney F.J., Lieberman M.D., Taylor S.E., Stretcher V.J. & Falk E.B. (2016). Self-affirmation activates brain systems associated with self-related processing and reward and is reinforced by future orientation. In *Social Cognitive and Affective Neuroscience*, Volume 11, Issue 4, 1 April 2016, pp 621–629, https://doi.org/10.1093/scan/nsv136

11 Harris P.S, Harris P.R. & Miles, W. (2017). Self-affirmation improves performance on tasks related to executive functioning. In *Journal of Experimental Social Psychology* Volume 70, May 2017, pp 281-285. www.sciencedirect.com/science/article/pii/S0022103116302840

12 Cohen, G.L. & Sherman, D.K. (2014). The psychology of change: Self-affirmation and social psychological intervention. *Annual Review of Psychology*, 65 (2014), pp 333-371, 10.1146/annurev-psych-010213-115137

Index

Published in 2019 by Murdoch Books,
an imprint of Allen & Unwin

Murdoch Books Australia
83 Alexander Street, Crows Nest NSW 2065
Phone: +61 (0)2 8425 0100
murdochbooks.com.au
info@murdochbooks.com.au

Murdoch Books UK
Ormond House, 26–27 Boswell Street,
London, WC1N 3JZ
Phone: +44 (0) 20 8785 5995
murdochbooks.co.uk
info@murdochbooks.co.uk

For Corporate Orders & Custom Publishing
contact our business development team at
salesenquiries@murdochbooks.com.au

Publisher: Kelly Doust
Design Manager and Designer: Madeleine Kane
Editorial Manager: Jane Price
Editor: Kylie Walker
Production Director: Lou Playfair

Photography: Amanda Prior, except pages 20, 23,
44, 106, 136 (left), 140, 173, 181, 215 by Chen Ryan;
41, 51 (top), 70 (top) by Bianca Cheah;
and 29 Bruno Martins; 40 Kunj Parekh and Daniel Straub
(images layered); 51 (bottom) Kenrick Mills; 72 (bottom)
Jacob Townsend; 76 Kumiko Shimizu; 79 Frank McKenna;
89 Jack Levick; 97 Alex Talmon; 112 Jordan McQueen;
113 Nathan Dumlao; 124 Simon Zachrisson; 136 (right)
Ruben Engel; 151 Max de Rohan Willner; 157 Jack Antal;
174 Valentin Polo; 185 Utsav Shah; 209 (left) Nordwood
Themes and (right) Aleksandra Boguslawskal; 211 Mel;
217 Davies Designs

Text © Kate Kendall
Design © Murdoch Books 2019
Photography © Amanda Prior, except pages 20, 23,
44, 106, 136 (left), 140, 173, 181, 215 © Chen Ryan;
pages 41, 51 (top), 70 (top) © Bianca Cheah;
and pages 29, 40, 51, 72 (bottom), 76, 79, 89, 97, 112,
113, 124, 136 (right), 151, 157, 174, 185, 209, 211, 217

ISBN 978 1 76052 412 8 Australia
ISBN 978 1 91163 215 3 UK

A cataloguing-in-publication entry is available from
the catalogue of the National Library of Australia at
nla.gov.au
A catalogue record for this book is available from the
British Library

Colour reproduction by Splitting Image Colour Studio
Pty Ltd, Clayton, Victoria

Printed by 1010 Printing Co Ltd, China

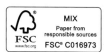